T0259456

Cardiopulmonary Resuscitation

Guest Editor

WANCHUN TANG, MD, Master CCM, FAHA

CRITICAL CARE CLINICS

www.criticalcare.theclinics.com

Consulting Editor
RICHARD W. CARLSON, MD, PhD

April 2012 • Volume 28 • Number 2

SAUNDERS an imprint of ELSEVIER, Inc.

W.B. SAUNDERS COMPANY
A Division of Elsevier Inc.

Elsevier Inc. • 1600 John F. Kennedy Blvd., • Suite 1800 • Philadelphia, Pennsylvania 19103-2899

http://www.theclinics.com

CRITICAL CARE CLINICS Volume 28, Number 2
April 2012 ISSN 0749-0704, ISBN-13: 978-1-4557-3845-8

Editor: Patrick Manley
Developmental Editor: Donald Mumford

© 2012 Elsevier Inc. All rights reserved.

This journal and the individual contributions contained in it are protected under copyright by Elsevier, and the following terms and conditions apply to their use:

Photocopying
Single photocopies of single articles may be made for personal use as allowed by national copyright laws. Permission of the Publisher and payment of a fee is required for all other photocopying, including multiple or systematic copying, copying for advertising or promotional purposes, resale, and all forms of document delivery. Special rates are available for educational institutions that wish to make photocopies for non-profit educational classroom use. For information on how to seek permission visit www.elsevier.com/permissions or call: (144) 1865 843830 (UK)/(11) 215 239 3804 (USA).

Derivative Works
Subscribers may reproduce tables of contents or prepare lists of articles including abstracts for internal circulation within their institutions. Permission of the Publisher is required for resale or distribution outside the institution. Permission of the Publisher is required for all other derivative works, including compilations and translations (please consult www.elsevier.com/permissions).

Electronic Storage or Usage
Permission of the Publisher is required to store or use electronically any material contained in this journal, including any article or part of an article (please consult www.elsevier.com/permissions). Except as outlined above, no part of this publication may be reproduced, stored in a retrieval system or transmitted in any form or by any means, electronic, mechanical, photocopying, recording or otherwise, without prior written permission of the Publisher.

Notice
No responsibility is assumed by the Publisher for any injury and/or damage to persons or property as a matter of products liability, negligence or otherwise, or from any use or operation of any methods, products, instructions or ideas contained in the material herein. Because of rapid advances in the medical sciences, in particular, independent verification of diagnoses and drug dosages should be made.

Although all advertising material is expected to conform to ethical (medical) standards, inclusion in this publication does not constitute a guarantee or endorsement of the quality or value of such product or of the claims made of it by its manufacturer.

Critical Care Clinics (ISSN: 0749-0704) is published quarterly by Elsevier Inc., 360 Park Avenue South, New York, NY 10010-1710. Months of issue are January, April, July, and October. Business and Editorial Offices: 1600 John F. Kennedy Blvd., Suite 1800, Philadelphia, PA 19103-2899. Customer Service Office: 6277 Sea Harbor Drive, Orlando, FL 32887-4800. Periodicals postage paid at New York, NY and additional mailing offices. Subscription prices are $193.00 per year for US individuals, $463.00 per year for US institution, $94.00 per year for US students and residents, $238.00 per year for Canadian individuals, $574.00 per year for Canadian institutions, $278.00 per year for international individuals, $574.00 per year for international institutions and $137.00 per year for Canadian and foreign students/residents. To receive student/resident rate, orders must be accompanied by name of affiliated institution, date of term, and the signature of program/residency coordinator on institution letterhead. Orders will be billed at individual rate until proof of status is received. Foreign air speed delivery is included in all *Clinics* subscription prices. All prices are subject to change without notice. POSTMASTER: Send address changes to *Critical Care Clinics,* Elsevier Periodicals Customer Service, 11830 Westline Industrial Drive, St. Louis, MO 63146. **Customer Service: 1-800-654-2452 (US). From outside of the US, call 1-314-447-8871. Fax: 1-314-447-8029. E-mail: journalscustomerservice-usa@elsevier.com (for print support) or journalsonlinesupport-usa@elsevier.com (for online support).**

Reprints. For copies of 100 or more of articles in this publication, please contact the Commercial Reprints Department, Elsevier Inc., 360 Park Avenue South, New York, NY 10010-1710. Tel.: 212-633-3813; Fax: 212-462-1935; E-mail: reprints@elsevier.com.

Critical Care Clinics is also published in Spanish by Editorial Inter-Medica, Junin 917, 1er A, 1113, Buenos Aires, Argentina.

Critical Care Clinics is covered in *MEDLINE/PubMed (Index Medicus), EMBASE/Excerpta Medica, Current Concepts/Clinical Medicine, ISI/BIOMED,* and *Chemical Abstracts.*

Printed and bound by CPI Group (UK) Ltd, Croydon, CR0 4YY

Transferred to Digital Print 2012

Contributors

CONSULTING EDITOR

RICHARD W. CARLSON, MD, PhD
Chairman Emeritus, Department of Medicine, Maricopa Medical Center; Director,
Medical Intensive Care Unit; Professor, University of Arizona College of Medicine;
Professor, Department of Medicine, Mayo Graduate School of Medicine, Phoenix,
Arizona

GUEST EDITOR

WANCHUN TANG, MD, Master CCM, FAHA
Professor, The Weil Institute of Critical Care Medicine, Rancho Mirage; The Keck
School of Medicine of the University of Southern California, Los Angeles, California

AUTHORS

LANCE B. BECKER, MD
Professor of Emergency Medicine; Director, Center for Resuscitation Science; Perelman
School of Medicine, University of Pennsylvania, Philadelphia, Pennsylvania

DAVID D. BERG, MD
Internal Medicine Resident, The Brigham and Women's Hospital and Harvard Medical
School, Boston, Massachusetts

ROBERT A. BERG, MD, FAHA, FCCM
Russell Raphaely Endowed Chair and Chief, Critical Care Medicine, The Children's
Hospital of Philadelphia; Professor of Anesthesiology and Critical Care, Perelman
School of Medicine, University of Pennsylvania, Philadelphia, Pennsylvania

MANUEL BOLLER, Dr MED. VET, MTR
Senior Research Investigator Critical Care and Anesthesia, School of Veterinary
Medicine, University of Pennsylvania, Philadelphia, Pennsylvania

MATTHIAS DERWALL, MD
Resident, Department of Anesthesiology, University Hospital Rheinisch-Westflische
Technische Hochschule Aachen, Aachen, Germany

MICHAEL FRIES, MD, PhD
Senior Staff Member, Department of Surgical Intensive Care, University Hospital
Rheinisch-Westflische Technische Hochschule Aachen, Aachen, Germany

DAVID F. GAIESKI, MD
Assistant Professor of Emergency Medicine; Clinical Director, Center for Resuscitation
Science; Perelman School of Medicine, University of Pennsylvania, Philadelphia, Pennsylvania

RAÚL J. GAZMURI, MD, PhD, FCCM
Chief, Section of Critical Care Medicine, Resuscitation Institute at Rosalind Franklin
University of Medicine and Science; Chief, Section of Critical Care Medicine, Medical
Service, Captain James A. Lovell Federal Health Care Center, North Chicago, Illinois

HENRY HALPERIN, MD, MA, FAHA, FHRS
Johns Hopkins University, Baltimore, Maryland

ERIK P. HESS, MD, MSc
Division of Emergency Medicine Research, Department of Emergency Medicine, Mayo Clinic College of Medicine; Knowledge and Evaluation Research Unit, Mayo Clinic, Rochester, Minnesota

KARL B. KERN, MD
Professor and Chief, Section of Cardiology, University of Arizona, Sarver Heart Center, Tucson, Arizona

SACHIN KUMAR, MD
Section of Cardiology, University of Arizona, Sarver Heart Center, Tucson, Arizona

YONGQIN LI, PhD
Assistant Professor, The Weil Institute of Critical Care Medicine, Rancho Mirage, California

ELMER MURDOCK, MD
Section of Cardiology, University of Arizona, Sarver Heart Center, Tucson, Arizona

JEEJABAI RADHAKRISHNAN, PhD
Research Assistant Professor, Director of the Molecular Laboratory and Associate Laboratory Manager, Resuscitation Institute at Rosalind Franklin University of Medicine and Science, North Chicago, Illinois

JASON A. STAMM, MD
Associate, Division of Pulmonary and Critical Care Medicine, Geisinger Medical Center, Danville, Pennsylvania

PETTER ANDREAS STEEN, MD, PhD
Professor of Medicine, University of Oslo; Prehospital Center, Oslo University Hospital, Oslo, Norway

RAJKUMAR K. SUGUMARAN, MD
Section of Cardiology, University of Arizona, Sarver Heart Center, Tucson, Arizona

SHIJIE SUN, MD
The Weil Institute of Critical Care Medicine, Rancho Mirage; The Keck School of Medicine of the University of Southern California, Los Angeles, California

KJETIL SUNDE, MD, PhD
Professor of Medicine, University of Oslo; Department of Anesthesiology, Oslo University Hospital, Oslo, Norway

WANCHUN TANG, MD, Master CCM, FAHA
Professor, The Weil Institute of Critical Care Medicine, Rancho Mirage; The Keck School of Medicine of the University of Southern California, Los Angeles, California

YINLUN WENG, MD
The Weil Institute of Critical Care Medicine, Rancho Mirage, California

ROGER D. WHITE, MD
Division of Cardiovascular Diseases, Department of Internal Medicine, Mayo Clinic College of Medicine; Medical Director, City of Rochester Early Defibrillation Program, Rochester, Minnesota

Contents

There are currently no data showing that vasopressor use during cardiac arrest improves neurologically intact survival. Epinephrine, both regular and high-dose, seems to improve short-term outcome but not long-term outcome. Vasopressin is an acceptable alternative to epinephrine. Researchers should be encouraged to continue experimental and clinical research on drugs and search for alternatives to epinephrine and vasopressin.

Optimizing the timing of defibrillation is of great importance in determining whether patients should receive immediate defibrillation versus delayed shock attempts with alternate therapies such as cardiopulmonary resuscitation (CPR) during cardiac arrest. Ventricular fibrillation (VF) waveforms change over time, and CPR exhibits predictable defibrillation success. Over the last few decades, many quantitative techniques have been developed to analyze VF waveforms to obtain more information about the state of the myocardium and the probability of successful defibrillation. This article summarizes the basics, the implications, and the limitations of analyzing the VF waveform for optimizing the timing of defibrillation during CPR.

Emergency cardiopulmonary bypass (ECPB) is advanced resuscitation strategy for patients with refractory cardiac arrest or cardiogenic shock unresponsive to traditional medical interventions. By diverting blood flow to an extracorporeal heart and lung system capable of providing full cardiac output, ECPB can provide blood flow and gas exchange when the patient has no capability of sustaining these functions intrinsically. Application of this method extends the time window for successful interventions to correct the underlying pathophysiology leading to arrest or shock. The authors define terms and concepts, provide a brief history of the method, give the rationale for its use, provide supporting evidence, and describe the most important clinical trials.

Mild therapeutic hypothermia (32°C–34°C) has been shown to improve survival and neurologic outcomes after sudden cardiac arrest in clinical studies. Its use is recommended by the American Heart Association for unconscious adult patients with spontaneous circulation after out-of-hospital ventricular fibrillation. It decreases cerebral metabolism and protects the brain after ischemia by reduction of brain metabolism, attenuation of neuroexcitotoxic cascade, abolition of reactive oxygen species, and inhibition of apoptosis. This article addresses the mechanism of neuroprotection, phases of hypothermia, and noninvasive and invasive cooling methods.

Successful resuscitation from cardiac arrest requires reestablishment of aerobic metabolism by reperfusion of tissues that have been deprived of oxygen for variable times. However, reperfusion concomitantly activates pathogenic mechanisms known as "reperfusion injury." Mitochondria play a critical role as effectors and targets of such injury. Mitochondrial injury compromises oxidative phosphorylation and prompts release of cytochrome *c* to the cytosol and bloodstream, where it correlates with severity of injury. Novel and clinically relevant strategies to protect mitochondrial bioenergetic function are expected to attenuate injury at the time of reperfusion and enhance organ viability, ultimately improving resuscitation and survival from cardiac arrest.

Neurologic dysfunction accounts for the majority of deaths in cardiac arrest survivors. Hence, improving the viability of cerebral nervous tissues represents the key challenge post cardiac arrest. Mild therapeutic hypothermia has been proven to ameliorate cerebral ischemia-reperfusion injury and is therefore the gold standard in postarrest care. Several neuroprotective drugs have been tested with much less encouraging results. These include hydrogen sulfide, xenon, and erythropoietin, Clinical trials are under way to learn whether these novel treatments will translate into measurable improvement. In addition, devices to improve myocardial and cerebral perfusion during and after cardiopulmonary resuscitation are being tested.

The vast majority of patients with out-of-hospital cardiac arrest have underlying coronary artery disease. Acute coronary ischemia is a common trigger for out-of-hospital ventricular fibrillation cardiac arrest. Often, culprit lesions can be readily identified during coronary angiography immediately after resuscitation. Coronary angiography after successful resuscitation should be done whenever a cardiac cause for the arrest is suspected. Early coronary angiography combined with mild therapeutic hypothermia is the best strategy for improving long-term neurologically intact survival in those successfully resuscitated. Cardiac arrest centers seem to be the best option for providing more cardiac arrest victims with aggressive postresuscitation care.

Jason A. Stamm

Edited by Kenneth E. Wood

Outcomes in acute pulmonary embolism (PE) are dictated by both patient factors and the hemodynamic consequences of pulmonary thromboembolism. Risk stratification in acute PE can be performed via clinical scoring systems, biomarkers, and imaging studies, including transthoracic echocardiography and CT angiography. Furthermore, there is a growing literature on the combination of risk stratification methods to better estimate outcomes. Whereas the negative predictive value for adverse events is high for many risk prediction tools, positive predictive value for all of these techniques, except in those patients who present in cardiogenic shock, remains low.

THE CLINICS ARE NOW AVAILABLE ONLINE!
Access your subscription at:
www.theclinics.com

Preface

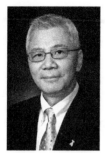

Wanchun Tang, MD, Master CCM
Guest Editor

The current disappointing outcome of cardiopulmonary resuscitation after sudden death reflects not only the constraints in implementation but also, in my opinion, the still primitive knowledge of the pathophysiology of cardiac arrest and the implication for resuscitation. Surprisingly, there is a paucity of research and research support. Such a fact, in part, reflects the lack of incentive to support such research. The perception of many, in both the professional and the lay communities, is that CPR is a "settled issue" that requires little or no additional research. Although the American Heart Association has always cautioned in each of the *Guidelines of CPR* otherwise, this perception of a settled issue continues.

Like science more generally, medical science usually advances at an escalating pace only when there is focus on unresolved challenges of large magnitudes. The disappointing statistics that have disclosed little or no improvement in outcome in the more than 50 years since modern CPR was introduced notwithstanding, the science has progressed but little in the absence of such a focus by the profession, by the public, and by the government. To illustrate the potential benefits, an improvement in outcome of CPR from the current approximately 5% national survival rate to as little as 20% would rescue more than two times the number of annual fatalities from automobile accidents.

This issue of *Critical Care Clinics* presents some of the major advances in the science of cardiopulmonary and cerebral resuscitation and is written by the internationally recognized experts in the field. I would like to express my sincere appreciation to those experts who contributed so richly to this issue. The subjects of this issue literally deal with life and death, death without warning, and death that occurs in out-of-hospital victims without terminal illnesses. It is very challenging to study victims under these conditions. The restraints are practical, ethical, and legal. In the absence of secure data on patients, a large part of the current knowledge and practices is based on experimental studies in animals. Although we appreciate that the guidelines of the American Heart Association may be the best reference to standards of practice, these, nevertheless, represent consensus often without secure evidence based on controlled studies. I am confident, however, that it will be advances

Crit Care Clin 28 (2012) xi–xiii
doi:10.1016/j.ccc.2012.01.001
0749-0704/12/$ – see front matter © 2012 Elsevier Inc. All rights reserved.

in science and, specifically, better objective data on victims that will account for improved outcomes.

The individual viewpoints of the authors were in each instance respected. Accordingly, the content of this issue is not constrained by a peer consensus. I would, therefore, alert the reader that, in some instances, the content differs significantly and understandably from published American Heart Association guidelines.

Wanchun Tang, MD, Master CCM
The Weil Institute of Critical Care Medicine
35-100 Bob Hope Drive
Rancho Mirage, CA 92270, USA

E-mail address:
drsheart@aol.com

Dedication

To the research team of the Weil Institute of Critical Care Medicine.

Automated External Defibrillation

Erik P. Hess, MD, MSc[a,b], Roger D. White, MD[c,d],*

KEYWORDS

- Defibrillators • Emergency medical services
- Out-of-hospital cardiac arrest • Sudden cardiac death

Automated external defibrillators (AEDs) are portable electronic devices designed to identify and defibrillate life-threatening arrhythmias in cardiac arrest victims. The primary application of AEDs is to treat ventricular fibrillation (VF) and pulseless ventricular tachycardia (VT) by operators with limited formal training in cardiac rhythm identification. AEDs use visual and voice prompts to guide both lay rescuers and health care professionals with infrequent contact with cardiac arrest victims through the process of providing rapid, effective cardiopulmonary resuscitation (CPR), rhythm identification, and early defibrillation of VF/VT in cardiac arrest victims.

HISTORY OF AUTOMATED EXTERNAL DEFIBRILLATION

In cardiac arrest victims, provision of high-quality CPR and early defibrillation are critical to survival. One model suggests that for each minute that passes between the time of collapse and defibrillation, survival in witnessed VF out-of-hospital cardiac arrest (OHCA) decreases by 7% to 10%.[1] When effective CPR is delivered, the decrement in survival over time becomes more gradual, averaging 3% to 4% each minute from collapse to defibrillation.[1–3] Moreover, if defibrillation can be provided within 5 to 10 minutes of arrest, many victims can survive the event neurologically intact.[4,5] With the introduction of hypothermia in care after arrest, neurologic outcomes may be improved to an even greater degree.

AEDs were originally developed as a strategy to reduce time to defibrillation and thereby increase survival in VF/VT cardiac arrest. Rather than wait for trained

[a] Division of Emergency Medicine Research, Department of Emergency Medicine, Mayo Clinic College of Medicine, 200 First Street SW, Rochester, MN 55905, USA
[b] Knowledge and Evaluation Research Unit, Mayo Clinic, 200 First Street SW, Rochester, MN 55905, USA
[c] Department of Anesthesiology and Division of Cardiovascular Diseases, Department of Internal Medicine, Mayo Clinic College of Medicine, 200 First Street SW, Rochester, MN 55905, USA
[d] City of Rochester Early Defibrillation Program, 200 First Street SW, Rochester, MN 55905, USA
* Corresponding author. Department of Anesthesiology and Division of Cardiovascular Diseases, Department of Internal Medicine, Mayo Clinic College of Medicine, 200 First Street SW, Rochester, MN 55905.
E-mail address: white.roger@mayo.edu

Crit Care Clin 28 (2012) 143–153
doi:10.1016/j.ccc.2011.10.009
0749-0704/12/$ – see front matter © 2012 Elsevier Inc. All rights reserved.

providers to arrive on-scene before intervening, AEDs provided a means for lay rescuers to provide defibrillation while trained health professionals were en route. Diack and colleagues described the first "automatic resuscitator" in 1979.[6] Referred to as the "Heart Aid," this 19-pound, portable, battery-powered device was capable of sensing two vital signs—heart beat and respiration rate—from which VF, asystole, or other nonarrest conditions were diagnosed. Once the device rendered an auto-mated diagnosis, a defibrillatory shock, pacing impulse, or no impulse was subse-quently delivered. As reliable rhythm identification algorithms had not yet been sufficiently developed at this stage, these investigators used a sensor to detect other signs of life not currently detected on modern AEDs—respiration—that was attached to an oropharyngeal airway. This sensor prevented the delivery of a shock as long as an air stream was detected over the tongue. This device was also unique in that it provided defibrillation through two electrodes, one of which was attached to the tongue and the other to the chest. Jaggarao and colleagues reported the first successful use of the Heart Aid by ambulance staff in 1982.[7] Cummins further demonstrated the safety and accuracy of this AED when used by paramedic staff to defibrillate OHCA victims in King County, Washington.[8] Eisenberg and colleagues reported increased cardiac arrest survival when emergency medical technicians were trained to used AEDs.[9] In 1982 Weaver and coworkers reported that initial shocks with 175 joules using a monophasic damped sine waveform (MDS) were as effective as shocks delivering 320 joules.[10] From these observations an automated external defibrillator was developed (LifePak 100, Physio-Control Corp, Redmond, WA, USA) that discharged nonescalating 180-joule MDS shocks. This was a major advance in automated defibrillator technology and also in both size and weight (2.5 kg). Efficacy with this device in terminating VF was documented by Weaver and colleagues.[11] Subsequently Weaver demonstrated improved neurologic recovery when AEDs were added to the armamentarium of basic life support (BLS)-trained first responders.[12] As efficacy data continued to accrue, firefighters[11,13,14] and police personnel[15] were subsequently equipped and trained to use AEDs. As the science supporting use of AEDs matured, it became clear that lay responders would play a vital role in improving survival in OHCA, and defibrillator manufacturers set out to develop portable devices that required minimal training to use effectively.

AED LIMITATIONS AND THE UNITED STATES FOOD AND DRUG ADMINISTRATION

Owing to rapidly accumulating evidence supporting use of AEDs in the prehospital setting, several major national and international agencies, including the American Heart Association,[16] the American College of Emergency Physicians,[17] the National Association of EMS physicians,[18] the Citizen CPR Foundation,[19] and others began to recommend use of AEDs as a critical component in early defibrillation. Shortly thereafter the US Food and Drug Administration (FDA) issued a safety alert in January 1994 regarding AEDs manufactured by Laerdal Manufacturing Corporation. The safety alert listed three main problems with two models of their devices: (1) failure to consistently shock VF; (2) delivery of an inappropriate shock to a non-VF rhythm; and (3) component failures. Two weeks after issuing the safety alert, the FDA filed a federal lawsuit, *United States v Laerdal Manufacturing Corporation*. The safety alert and trial resulted from two cases reported by the manufacturer to the FDA, as required by law. These two cases presented by the FDA—one in which the AED failed to shock VF and one in which the AED inappropriately shocked sinus rhythm—were used to support their claim that AEDs were a public health hazard. This allegation occurred despite several studies[20–22] indicating excellent but not perfect performance of AEDs in defibrillating VF in cardiac arrest. Given the large body of evidence supporting the critical contribution of AEDs to early defibrillation and survival in cardiac arrest, resuscitation experts and prominent national and international organizations continued to recommend the use of AEDs.[22]

On January 25, 2010 the FDA convened a Circulatory Systems Devices Panel to determine the requirements for manufacturers who design new modifications or improvements in AED design and function. The FDA classifies devices into one of three categories: Class I are low-risk devices for which general controls such as registration and listing with the FDA, compliance with quality system regulations, and reporting of adverse events are required. Class II devices are moderate-risk devices for which special controls in addition to general controls are required to provide assurance of safety and effectiveness. Types of special controls include performance standards, postmarket surveillance, patient registries, specific testing (bench, animal, and clinical), and other requirements. For example, if a device were to have a new mechanical component, a manufacturer would need to identify the required bench test, including a test protocol and acceptance criteria, to assess the mechanical integrity of the device. A class II device would likely require submission of a 510(k) application before marketing. Class III devices are the highest risk devices. These devices warrant additional controls and rigorous testing to determine the safety and effectiveness of a device. Class III devices require submission of a premarket approval application (PMA) to the FDA before making a device commercially available. The PMA application is the most rigorous standard and requires demonstration of the greatest degree of evidence of safety and effectiveness relative to the 510(k) application.

Before the convening of this panel, AEDs were classified as class III devices, the most high risk type, but submission of PMA applications for FDA approval was not required. Rather, AED manufacturers were required to submit 510(k) applications for consideration of FDA approval. The purpose of the panel was to reconfirm the classification of AEDs as class III devices, and thus require submission of PMA applications, or to reclassify them to class II, subject only to premarket notification, or 510(k) applications.

The FDA panel conducted an independent, comprehensive, systematic review of the literature, a review of the performance testing currently required for PMAs, an analysis of medical device reports (MDRs) as related to engineering design and quality management, and an analysis of AED recalls submitted from 2005 to 2010.

When conducting performance testing, the FDA conducts an analysis comparing the differences between a new (or modified device) and the device currently on the market ("predicate" device). Previous performance testing had involved bench testing (eg, engineering testing such as defibrillation waveform testing in the form of oscilloscope captures and waveform parameters measurements), animal testing (when a new defibrillation waveform is not identical to the predicate waveform but the difference is not significant enough to require clinical testing), premarket clinical testing (when a new defibrillation waveform is significantly different from a preexisting waveform or when new user interfaces such as device screens, control dials, or voice prompts are developed, requiring human factors testing), and, on rare occasion, postmarket clinical testing.

A review of the MDRs from 2005 to 2010 revealed 23,591 device reports. Although each MDR event did not necessarily represent events that occurred during device use (some may represent AED self-diagnostics when no patient was involved), this number is substantial. Among the 23,591 MDRs, in only 7916 (33.5%) did the manufacturer follow-up the MDR and submit the follow-up report to the FDA. Finally, it was noted that the total number of MDRs substantially increased over the 5-year period and that the increase was evenly distributed among event types (eg, death, injury, device malfunction, other).

Review of manufacturer recalls over the time period identified 68 recalls. The recalls were classified into class I (in which there is a reasonable probability that exposure to the AED caused serious adverse health consequences or death), class II (exposure to the AED may have caused temporary or reversible adverse health consequences or the likelihood of serious adverse health consequences is remote), and class III. Among the 68 recalls, 17 were classified as class I, 48 as class II, 1 was classified as class III, and 2 were considered safety alerts. In root cause analyses of the recalls, the FDA determined that with the exception of one recall related to the distribution of a device without a 510(k), the remaining recalls were likely related to product defects resulting from failure of manufacturers' quality management systems.

Based on the need to optimize the sensitivity and specificity of arrhythmia detection algorithms and shock delivery during CPR, the panel noted that optimiza tion of electrical therapy during resuscitation required high-quality performance data, optimally in the form of prospective randomized clinical trials. In addition, based on review of the MDR reports and recalls over the 5-year study period, the panel recommended improved premarket and postmarket review of AEDs. No final decision has been made by the FDA on reclassification. Conflicts with the FDA regarding AEDs have been described in a previous evaluation referring to "confrontation without comprehension."[23] The next section reviews AED clinical applications.

CURRENT CLINICAL APPLICATIONS OF AEDS

Clinical applications are based on recommendations and evidence supporting the following: integration of CPR with AED use, development of lay rescuer AED programs to improve survival rates from OHCA, and strategic placement of AEDs to improve cardiac arrest survival.

As time passes in VF, stores of myocardial oxygen and metabolic substrates become depleted, decreasing the effectiveness of delivered shocks. Provision of an initial period of CPR before defibrillation supplies much needed oxygen and substrates, thus increasing shock effectiveness and the likelihood that a perfusing rhythm will be restored. This physiologic rationale underlies treatment approaches and recommendations regarding integration of CPR with AED use such that delays to either the start of CPR or provision of defibrillation are minimized.

Fig. 1 illustrates the integration of CPR with AED use. Immediately after a witnessed collapse, the rescuer should perform BLS interventions consisting of confirming unresponsiveness by tapping the victim on the shoulder and shouting at the victim.[24] If the victim does not respond, the next step is to activate the emergency medical services (EMS) system. If an AED is immediately available, the rescuer should provide defibrillation as soon as possible. If no AED is immediately available and the time from activation of EMS to arrival of care providers is greater than 4 to 5 minutes, 1.5 to 3 minutes of CPR can be provided before assessment for a shockable rhythm. Treatment should then proceed as indicated according to the updated ACLS 2010 AHA treatment algorithm.[25] In unwitnessed OHCA, lay responders or EMS personnel should perform BLS interventions and immediately initiate CPR. CPR should be performed while the AED is being prepared for use. There is insufficient evidence to determine if 1.5 to 3 minutes of CPR should be performed before defibrillation in unwitnessed OHCA.[26,27]

To increase survival in sudden cardiac arrest, lay rescuer AED programs should be developed with the goal of increasing the frequency and quality of bystander CPR and decreasing the time to defibrillation. In the Ontario Prehospital Advanced Life Support

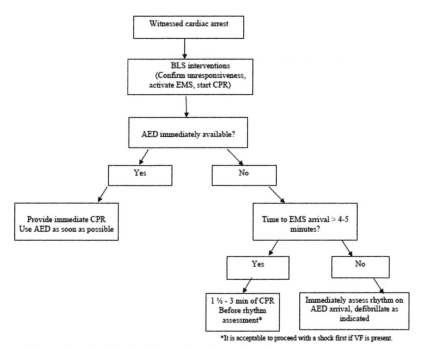

Fig. 1. Integration of CPR with AED use in witnessed cardiac arrest.

study, which included 5638 OHCA victims from 17 cities, both bystander CPR and defibrillation in less than 8 minutes were strong independent predictors of survival. However, bystanders provided CPR before EMS arrival in only 15% of cases.[28] Reports of the rates of bystander CPR in other cities are also quite low.[29-31] One of the reported barriers to provision of bystander CPR is concern about potential disease transmission and disagreeable physical characteristics (eg, presence of vomitus, dentures, or blood or alcohol on the breath) related to performing mouth-to-mouth ventilation.[32,33] In an effort to increase the proportion of OHCA victims who receive bystander CPR, the AHA released a science advisory statement recommending hands-only CPR for lay rescuers before arrival of EMS.[34] Whether change from traditional to hands-only CPR results in increased rates of bystander CPR remains to be seen.

Several studies of lay rescuer AED programs have shown increased survival related to decreased time to defibrillation. Equipping police officers[15,35] and fire personnel[36] with AEDs and incorporating them into the emergency response is one approach that has been shown to decrease the time to defibrillation and increase survival in some settings. In the Public Access Defibrillation (PAD) study, a large prospective community-based multicenter trial, community units (eg, shopping malls and apartment complexes) were randomly assigned to an emergency response system in which lay volunteers were trained in CPR alone or in CPR and the use of AEDs.[37] The programs included a structured and planned emergency response, training of lay rescuers, and frequent retraining. These investigators observed that survival to hospital discharge doubled in community units randomized to CPR + AEDs. In another large population-based observational study of OHCA victims enrolled in the Resuscitation Outcomes Consortium epistry, it was observed that application of an AED was associated with nearly a doubling in survival (odds ratio [OR], 1.75; 95% confidence interval [CI], 1.23–2.50) after adjusting for known confounders in multivariable analyses.[38]

Survival from sudden cardiac arrest is greater when the arrest is witnessed and an AED is immediately available. This has been demonstrated in studies reporting impressive survival rates in airplanes,[39] casinos,[40] and airports.[41] Given these promising results, a logical consideration is whether placement of AEDs in homes would be associated with similar improvements in survival. In the Home Automated External Defibrillator Trial (HAT), 7001 patients who had previously suffered an anterior wall myocardial infarction but were not candidates for implantable cardioverter-defibrillator were randomized to either receiving an AED for home use or no AED.[42] These investigators observed that, compared to a standard emergency response, placement of an AED in homes did not increase survival.

Once a lay rescuer AED program has been established, it is important to implement processes of continuous quality improvement (CQI). To run an effective CQI program for OHCA, it is critical to develop processes to capture EMS-system, EMS-provider, and first responder performance and patient outcomes. This will enable EMS directors to orchestrate routine inspections of EMS system-level and provider-level performance, monitor the contribution of lay responders to the EMS response, and use critical postevent data to provide feedback to care providers to improve the quality of care delivered to OHCA victims.[43,44]

STRATEGIC PLACEMENT OF AEDS TO IMPROVE CARDIAC ARREST SURVIVAL

In a recent study correlating the location of cardiac arrest, the initial recorded rhythm, and the probability of survival, 84% of arrests occurred in a private or residential setting and 16% occurred in a public location.[45] Of the arrests that occurred in private or residential settings, 18% had VF or pulseless VT as the initial rhythm and 5% survived to hospital discharge. Of the arrests that occurred in public settings, 51% had VF/VT as the initial rhythm and 17% survived to hospital discharge.

These data have implications regarding the potential survival benefit of placing AEDs in specific locations. Although the vast majority of cardiac arrests occur in private or residential settings, results from the HAT trial indicate that placing AEDs in homes is not likely to improve survival. Evidence suggests that placement of AEDs in public locations, where arrests are likely to be witnessed, is the most effective strategy for improving survival in OHCA.

Where should PAD programs be developed and AEDs strategically placed? Previous studies suggest that airlines, airports, and casinos are public locations that will likely benefit from AEDs being available. Developing PAD programs for these niche areas, however, is not an effective approach to increase cardiac arrest survival in a community. Guidelines from the AHA recommend that AEDs be placed in locations in which at least one cardiac arrest occurs every 5 years.[46] A recent study in Copenhagen, Denmark described the use of a geographical information system to document the location of cardiac arrests and strategically place AEDs where arrests are likely to occur.[47] Results from this study support the feasibility and cost-effectiveness of placing AEDs in accordance with AHA recommendations.

RECENT DEVELOPMENTS

The deployment of AEDs in places in which they are most likely to be beneficial is an area of active study. It is evident from the HAT trial that placement of AEDs in the home does not have a major impact on survival from cardiac arrest, in large part because only a small number of arrests in homes are treatable with defibrillation. The study by Weisfeldt and colleagues[38] demonstrated the very low incidence of VF as the initial rhythm in the home when compared with public settings. In that study, only 22% of the arrests in homes presented in VF whereas in public settings the incidence of VF was 51%. In the study by Folke and colleagues,[48] the incidence of VF as the initial rhythm was 12.8% in residential locations and 38.1% in public locations. These data are consistent with the PAD trial relative to VF as the initial rhythm in public locations. Thus efforts to improve survival from cardiac arrest outside the hospital need to be directed toward identifying strategic public locations in which AED deployment has the maximum likelihood of benefit.

For several years clinical investigations have been directed toward analysis of the VF waveform with AED algorithms in an attempt to differentiate VF that has a high likelihood of benefitting with a shock as opposed to preceding the shock with a period of CPR with the intent that the CPR will better prepare the VF for an effective shock.[49–51] This technology is already incorporated in some AEDs and no doubt will be included in others as this development is pursued and perfected. The endpoint of all of these approaches is to identify VF that will transition to an organized rhythm with the potential of regaining a spontaneous circulation with a shock. These algorithms utilize several VF characteristics, including frequency, amplitude, conduction (VF slope), and the VF power spectrum.

AREAS OF ONGOING INVESTIGATION

All efforts in current and future research designs are intended to increase the likelihood that defibrillation shocks with AEDs will not only terminate VF but will also increase the frequency with which a functional organized rhythm is restored with the shock. Analysis of the rhythm while chest compressions are continuing without interruption is intended to maintain blood flow without the need for a pause for artifact-free rhythm analysis. Longer perishock and preshock pauses were shown in one study to be independently associated with a decrease in survival to discharge.[52] Defibrillator charging can be accomplished during ongoing chest compressions and thus decrease hands-off time.[53] Likewise there is interest in enabling shocks to be delivered while CPR is in progress, again to avoid the need to pause and thereby cease blood flow. The safety of shocking with CPR in progress is under investigation.[54–56]

Provision of CPR feedback during CPR is becoming common practice. Although most evidence supports benefit from reducing hands-off time during CPR, one study which shortened pauses during CPR and increased hands-on time did not observe an increase in survival to hospital admission.[57] It is likely that in the future this feedback will be driven by measures of perfusion rather than by somewhat arbitrary standards of CPR performance. Monitoring end-tidal carbon dioxide tension is an objective index of blood flow during CPR and can be used to guide CPR performance to maximize blood flow with chest compressions.[58–61]

Another area in which it is likely that future developments can be anticipated is in the analysis of the VF waveform in such a manner that the appropriate timing of a shock related to certain moments during ongoing VF and CPR can be exploited. There may be precise moments during VF when a shock is more likely to be effective than at others. One experimental study reported that defibrillation efficacy was maximal when the shock was delivered during the upstroke phase of mechanical chest compressions.[62]

Finally, geo-location of AEDs is likely to evolve. One possibility in this situation is that a signal could be delivered from an AED to cell phones to alert potential rescuers and thereby bring them to the cardiac arrest victim and the AED at that site. One pilot study assessed a Short Message Service (SMS) with which laypersons were alerted to proceed to patients with suspected out-of-hospital cardiac arrest and perform CPR and use an AED. This study described a program in which emergency medical services dispatch alerted citizens by sending SMS messages on their mobile phones.[63] More experience with this technology is needed but these early results are very encouraging.

SUMMARY

In conclusion, AEDs are low-energy portable electronic devices designed to treat VF and pulseless VT by operators with limited formal training in cardiac rhythm identification. AEDs are a key component of the BLS sequence and should be closely integrated with high-quality chest compressions such that delays in both the start of CPR and provision of defibrillation are minimized. Lay rescuer AED programs have been demonstrated to decrease the time to defibrillation and increase survival to hospital discharge in some settings. To optimally increase survival in OHCA, AEDs should be placed in public settings in which at least one cardiac arrest is expected to occur every 5 years. Several areas of ongoing investigation—such as automated VF waveform analysis, provision of feedback during CPR, geo-location of AEDs at the time of the arrest, and SMS mobile phone messaging—seek to further improve survival in victims of sudden cardiac arrest.

REFERENCES

1. Larsen MP, Eisenberg MS, Cummins RO, et al. Predicting survival from out-of-hospital cardiac arrest: a graphic model. Ann Emerg Med 1993;22(11):1652–8.
2. Valenzuela TD, Roe DJ, Cretin S, et al. Estimating effectiveness of cardiac arrest interventions: a logistic regression survival model. Circulation 1997;96(10):3308–13.
3. Stiell IG, Wells GA, Field B, et al. Advanced cardiac life support in out-of-hospital cardiac arrest. N Engl J Med 2004;351(7):647–56.
4. Cummins RO, Eisenberg MS, Hallstrom AP, et al. Survival of out-of-hospital cardiac arrest with early initiation of cardiopulmonary resuscitation. Am J Emerg Med 1985; 3(2):114–9.
5. Holmberg M, Holmberg S, Herlitz J. Effect of bystander cardiopulmonary resuscitation in out-of-hospital cardiac arrest patients in Sweden. Resuscitation 2000;47(1):59–70.
6. Diack AW, Welborn WS, Rullman RG, et al. An automatic cardiac resuscitator for emergency treatment of cardiac arrest. Med Instrum 1979;13(2):78–83.
7. Jaggarao NS, Heber M, Grainger R, et al. Use of an automated external defibrillator-pacemaker by ambulance staff. Lancet 1982;2(8289):73–5.
8. Cummins RO, Eisenberg M, Bergner L, et al. Sensitivity, accuracy, and safety of an automatic external defibrillator. Lancet 1984;2(8398):318–20.
9. Eisenberg MS, Copass MK, Hallstrom AP, et al. Treatment of out-of-hospital cardiac arrests with rapid defibrillation by emergency medical technicians. N Engl J Med 1980;302(25):1379–83.
10. Weaver WD, Cobb LA, Copass MK, et al. Ventricular defibrillation—a comparative trial using 175-J and 320-J shocks. N Engl J Med 1982;307(18):1101–6.
11. Weaver WD, Copass MK, Hill DL, et al. Cardiac arrest treated with a new automatic external defibrillator by out-of-hospital first responders. Am J Cardiol 1986;57(13): 1017–21.
12. Weaver WD, Copass MK, Bufi D, et al. Improved neurologic recovery and survival after early defibrillation. Circulation 1984;69(5):943–8.

13. Weaver WD, Hill D, Fahrenbruch CE, et al. Use of the automatic external defibrillator in the management of out-of-hospital cardiac arrest. N Engl J Med 1988;319(11): 661–6.
14. Shuster M, Keller JL. Effect of fire department first-responder automated defibrillation. Ann Emerg Med 1993;22(4):721–7.
15. White RD, Vukov LF, Bugliosi TF. Early defibrillation by police: initial experience with measurement of critical time intervals and patient outcome. Ann Emerg Med 1994; 23(5):1009–13.
16. Cummins RO, Thies W. Encouraging early defibrillation: the American Heart Association and automated external defibrillators. Ann Emerg Med 1990;19(11):1245–8.
17. McDowell R, Krohmer J, Spaite DW, et al. Guidelines for implementation of early defibrillation/automated external defibrillator programs. American College of Emergency Physicians. Ann Emerg Med 1993;22(4):740–1.
18. Paris PM. EMT-defibrillation: a recipe for saving lives. Am J Emerg Med 1988;6(3): 282–7.
19. Newman M. Defibrillation shakes the nation. Results of the JEMS 1988 National Early Defibrillation Study. JEMS 1989;14(1):50–6, 58–9.
20. Dickey W, Dalzell GW, Anderson JM, et al. The accuracy of decision-making of a semi-automatic defibrillator during cardiac arrest. Eur Heart J 1992;13(5):608–15.
21. Cummins RO, Stults KR, Haggar B, et al. A new rhythm library for testing automatic external defibrillators: performance of three devices. J Am Coll Cardiol 1988;11(3): 597–602.
22. Kellermann AL, Hackman BB, Dobyns P, et al. Engineering excellence: options to enhance firefighter compliance with standing orders for first-responder defibrillation. Ann Emerg Med 1993;22(8):1269–75.
23. Cummins RO, White RD, Pepe PE. Ventricular fibrillation, automatic external defibrillators, and the United States Food and Drug Administration: confrontation without comprehension. Ann Emerg Med 1995;26(5):621–31 [discussion: 632–4].
24. Berg RA, Hemphill R, Abella BS, et al. Part 5: Adult basic life support. Circulation 2010;122(18 Suppl 3):S685–S705.
25. Neumar RW, Otto CW, Link MS, et al. Part 8: adult advanced cardiovascular life support: 2010 American Heart Association Guidelines for Cardiopulmonary Resuscitation and Emergency Cardiovascular Care. Circulation 2010;122(18 Suppl 3):S729–67.
26. Koike S, Tanabe S, Ogawa T, et al. Immediate defibrillation or defibrillation after cardiopulmonary resuscitation. Prehosp Emerg Care 2011;15(3):393–400.
27. Simpson PM, Goodger MS, Bendall JC. Delayed versus immediate defibrillation for out-of-hospital cardiac arrest due to ventricular fibrillation: a systematic review and meta-analysis of randomised controlled trials. Resuscitation 2010;81(8):925–31.
28. Stiell IG, Wells GA, Field B, et al. Advanced cardiac life support in out-of-hospital cardiac arrest. N Engl J Med 2004;351(7):647–56.
29. Swor R, Khan I, Domeier R, et al. CPR training and CPR performance: do CPR-trained bystanders perform CPR? Acad Emerg Med 2006;13(6):596–601.
30. Lateef F, Anantharaman V. Bystander cardiopulmonary resuscitation in prehospital cardiac arrest patients in Singapore. Prehosp Emerg Care 2001;5(4):387–90.
31. SOS-KANTO study group. Cardiopulmonary resuscitation by bystanders with chest compression only (SOS-KANTO): an observational study. Lancet 2007;369(9565): 920–6.
32. McCormack AP, Damon SK, Eisenberg MS. Disagreeable physical characteristics affecting bystander CPR. Ann Emerg Med 1989;18(3):283–5.

33. Locke CJ, Berg RA, Sanders AB, et al. Bystander cardiopulmonary resuscitation. Concerns about mouth-to-mouth contact. Arch Intern Med 1995;155(9):938–43.

34. Sayre MR, Berg RA, Cave DM, et al. Hands-only (compression-only) cardiopulmonary resuscitation: a call to action for bystander response to adults who experience out-of-hospital sudden cardiac arrest: a science advisory for the public from the American Heart Association Emergency Cardiovascular Care Committee. Circulation 2008;117(16):2162–7.

35. White RD, Hankins DG, Bugliosi TF. Seven years' experience with early defibrillation by police and paramedics in an emergency medical services system. Resuscitation 1998;39(3):145–51.

36. White RD, Bunch TJ, Hankins DG. Evolution of a community-wide early defibrillation programme: experience over 13 years using police/fire personnel and paramedics as responders. Resuscitation 2005;65(3):279–83.

37. The Public Access Defibrillation Trial Investigators. Public-access defibrillation and survival after out-of-hospital cardiac arrest. N Engl J Med 2004;351(7):637–46.

38. Weisfeldt ML, Sitlani CM, Ornato JP, et al. Survival after application of automatic external defibrillators before arrival of the emergency medical system: evaluation in the resuscitation outcomes consortium population of 21 million. J Am Coll Cardiol 2010;55(16):1713–20.

39. Page RL, Joglar JA, Kowal RC, et al. Use of automated external defibrillators by a U.S. airline. N Engl J Med 2000;343(17):1210–6.

40. Valenzuela TD, Roe DJ, Nichol G, et al. Outcomes of rapid defibrillation by security officers after cardiac arrest in casinos. N Engl J Med 2000;343(17):1206–9.

41. Caffrey SL, Willoughby PJ, Pepe PE, et al. Public use of automated external defibrillators. N Engl J Med 2002;347(16):1242–7.

42. Bardy GH, Lee KL, Mark DB, et al. Home use of automated external defibrillators for sudden cardiac arrest. N Engl J Med 2008;358(17):1793–804.

43. Eisenberg M, White RD. The unacceptable disparity in cardiac arrest survival among American communities. Ann Emerg Med 2009;54(2):258–60.

44. Hess EP, White RD. Optimizing survival from out-of-hospital cardiac arrest. J Cardiovasc Electrophysiol 2010;21(5):590–5.

45. Weisfeldt ML, Everson-Stewart S, Sitlani C, et al. Ventricular tachyarrhythmias after cardiac arrest in public versus at home. N Engl J Med 2011;364(4):313–21.

46. Aufderheide T, Hazinski MF, Nichol G, et al. Community lay rescuer automated external defibrillation programs: key state legislative components and implementation strategies: a summary of a decade of experience for healthcare providers, policymakers, legislators, employers, and community leaders from the American Heart Association Emergency Cardiovascular Care Committee, Council on Clinical Cardiology, and Office of State Advocacy. Circulation 2006;113(9):1260–70.

47. Folke F, Lippert FK, Nielsen L Sr, et al. Location of cardiac arrest in a city center. Circulation 2009;120(6):510–7.

48. Folke F, Gislason GH, Lippert FK, et al. Differences between out-of-hospital cardiac arrest in residential and public locations and implications for public-access defibrillation. Circulation 2010;122(6):623–30.

49. Eftestol T, Sunde K, Ole Aase S, et al. Predicting outcome of defibrillation by spectral characterization and nonparametric classification of ventricular fibrillation in patients with out-of-hospital cardiac arrest. Circulation 2000;102(13):1523–9.

50. Eftestol T, Wik L, Sunde K, et al. Effects of cardiopulmonary resuscitation on predictors of ventricular fibrillation defibrillation success during out-of-hospital cardiac arrest. Circulation 2004;110(1):10–5.

51. Young C, Bisera J, Gehman S, et al. Amplitude spectrum area: measuring the probability of successful defibrillation as applied to human data. Crit Care Med 2004;32(9 Suppl):S356–8.
52. Cheskes S, Schmicker RH, Christenson J, et al. Perishock pause: an independent predictor of survival from out-of-hospital shockable cardiac arrest. Circulation 2011; 124(1):58–66.
53. Edelson DP, Robertson-Dick BJ, Yuen TC, et al. Safety and efficacy of defibrillator charging during ongoing chest compressions: a multi-center study. Resuscitation 2010;81(11):1521–6.
54. Lloyd MS, Heeke B, Walter PF, et al. Hands-on defibrillation: an analysis of electrical current flow through rescuers in direct contact with patients during biphasic external defibrillation. Circulation 2008;117(19):2510–4.
55. Hoke RS, Heinroth K, Trappe HJ, et al. Is external defibrillation an electric threat for bystanders? Resuscitation 2009;80(4):395–401.
56. Perkins GD, Lockey AS. Defibrillation—safety versus efficacy. Resuscitation 2008; 79(1):1–3.
57. Jost D, Degrange H, Verret C, et al. DEFI 2005: a randomized controlled trial of the effect of automated external defibrillator cardiopulmonary resuscitation protocol on outcome from out-of-hospital cardiac arrest. Circulation 2010;121(14):1614–22.
58. Asplin BR, White RD. Prognostic value of end-tidal carbon dioxide pressures during out-of-hospital cardiac arrest. Ann Emerg Med 1995;25(6):756–61.
59. Kolar M, Krizmaric M, Klemen P, et al. Partial pressure of end-tidal carbon dioxide successful predicts cardiopulmonary resuscitation in the field: a prospective observational study. Crit Care 2008;12(5):R115.
60. Weil MH. Partial pressure of end-tidal carbon dioxide predicts successful cardiopulmonary resuscitation in the field. Crit Care 2008;12(6):90.
61. White RD, Goodman BW, Svoboda MA. Neurologic recovery following prolonged out-of-hospital cardiac arrest with resuscitation guided by continuous capnography. Mayo Clin Proc 2011;86(6):544–8.
62. Li Y, Yu T, Ristagno G, et al. The optimal phasic relationship between synchronized shock and mechanical chest compressions. Resuscitation 2010;81(6):724–9.
63. Scholten AC, van Manen JG, van der Worp WE, et al. Early cardiopulmonary resuscitation and use of automated external defibrillators by laypersons in out-of-hospital cardiac arrest using an SMS alert service. Resuscitation 2011;82(10): 1273–8.

When Should Rescue Breathing Be Removed From the ABCs of CPR?

David D. Berg, MD[a], Robert A. Berg, MD, FCCM[b],*

KEYWORDS

- Cardiac arrest • Cardiopulmonary resuscitation
- Rescue breathing • Ventilation • Heart arrest

Cardiac arrest is a major public health problem and a leading cause of death in the United States.[1] Nearly 300,000 Americans sustain out-of-hospital cardiac arrests (OHCAs) each year, and cardiopulmonary resuscitation (CPR) is provided by emergency medical professionals for approximately 175,000 of these OHCA victims each year.[2] Although prompt initiation of bystander CPR substantially improves the chances of survival from OHCA, most cardiac arrest victims do not receive bystander CPR.[3] In-hospital cardiac arrests (IHCAs) and CPR are also relatively common. A recent study has established that CPR is provided for approximately 200,000 hospitalized patients each year.[4]

Fifty years ago, Kouwenhoven and colleagues[5] demonstrated that "closed chest cardiac massage" resulted in successful return of spontaneous circulation for 20 consecutive patients with IHCAs. Their animal studies showed that closed chest cardiac massage (without rescue breathing) was an effective technique to maintain circulation of dogs in ventricular fibrillation (VF) for up to 30 minutes, thereby allowing successful defibrillation and return of spontaneous circulation. Therefore, the initial patients in this clinical series received chest compressions without artificial respiration. Artificial respiration was soon added to closed chest cardiac massage because of the presumed need for adequate oxygenation and ventilation. The new bundle was taught as the ABCs of CPR.

Financial disclosures: Dr Robert A. Berg has had relevant research grants from National Heart, Lung, and Blood Institute, The American Heart Association, and The Arizona Disease Control Research Commission. Dr David D. Berg and Dr Robert A. Berg report no financial conflicts of interest.

[a] The Brigham and Women's Hospital and Harvard Medical School, Internal Medicine Residency Office, 75 Francis Street, Boston, MA 02115, USA
[b] Department of Anesthesiology and Critical Care Medicine, The Children's Hospital of Philadelphia and The University of Pennsylvania Perelman School of Medicine, 34th Street and Civic Center Boulevard, 7 South Tower, Room #7C26, Philadelphia, PA 19104, USA
* Corresponding author.
E-mail address: bergra@email.chop.edu

Crit Care Clin 28 (2012) 155–165
doi:10.1016/j.ccc.2011.12.001
0749-0704/12/$ – see front matter © 2012 Elsevier Inc. All rights reserved.

WHAT IS THE VALUE OF HANDS-ONLY CPR?

Animal Studies Regarding the Need for Assisted Ventilation During CPR for Ventricular Fibrillation

Chandra and colleagues[6] showed that dogs in VF could maintain arterial oxygen saturation greater than 90% for more than 4 minutes of CPR. Many swine studies over the last 20 years have shown that chest compressions alone (hands-only CPR) are as effective as chest compressions plus assisted ventilation for VF cardiac arrests.[7-13] These results include studies with chest compressions for up to 12 minutes, chest compressions in the setting of induced acute myocardial infarction with coronary artery obstruction, and chest compressions with clamping of the endotracheal tube designed to simulate an obstructed airway during CPR for VF. Importantly, hands-only CPR is more effective than chest compression plus rescue breathing in realistic animal models of single-rescuer bystander CPR with the typical 16 seconds of interruptions in chest compressions associated with moving from the chest to the head, providing two rescue breaths with a good mouth-to-mouth seal, and returning to the side of the chest to restart chest compressions.[13-19]

Why Is Assisted Ventilation Not Necessary for VF?

Because oxygenation and ventilation are clearly important for survival from cardiac arrest, why is assisted ventilation ("rescue breathing") not necessary in these animal models of VF cardiac arrest? Immediately after an acute fibrillatory cardiac arrest, aortic oxygen and carbon dioxide concentrations do not vary from the prearrest state because there is no blood flow during untreated VF, and aortic oxygen consumption is minimal. Therefore, when chest compressions are initiated, blood flowing from the aorta to the coronary and cerebral circulation provides adequate oxygenation at an acceptable pH. At that time, myocardial and cerebral oxygen delivery are limited by blood flow rather than oxygen content. Importantly, the lung at the time of VF is a reservoir with substantial oxygen and limited carbon dioxide. During chest compressions, the oxygen reservoir in the lungs provides adequate oxygenation of the limited pulmonary blood flow, and the lungs provide a reservoir for unloading carbon dioxide. Therefore, arterial partial pressure of oxygen, partial pressure of carbon dioxide, and pH can be adequate for several minutes even with airway obstruction. In addition, animals (and humans) have substantial active ventilation (gasping) during CPR, which provides additional gas exchange.[20,21] Finally, when the airway is not occluded, significant chest compression–induced gas exchange can occur because of the negative intrathoracic pressure associated with chest recoil in the relaxation phase of external chest compressions. Assisted ventilation was not necessary in many fibrillatory arrest experiments because arterial oxygen saturation and pH were adequate with chest compressions alone; consequently, myocardial and cerebral oxygen delivery were adequate with chest compressions alone. Assisted ventilation may become rate-limiting in animal VF CPR investigations when CPR for VF is prolonged and/or when the animal has received paralytic agents that prevent gasping and increase the tendency for progressive atelectasis (ie, decreasing functional residual capacity, thereby decreasing residual oxygen in the lung available for gas exchange).[22] Bottom line: oxygenation and ventilation are important, but rescue breathing is not necessary for adequate oxygenation and ventilation during the initial minutes of CPR for VF.

Observational Studies for Hands-Only Bystander CPR

Several observational cohort studies from Belgium, Japan, Singapore, Norway and Sweden suggest that hands-only bystander CPR is as effective as chest compressions

Table 1			
Observational studies of bystander CPR for OHCA: hands-only CPR versus conventional CPR			
Location	Population (N)	Primary End Point	Hands-Only CPR Vs Conventional CPR RR [95% CI][a]
Belgium[23]	All OHCA with good quality CPR (3053)	14-day survival	17/116 (15%) vs 71/443 (16%) 0.91 [0.56–1.49]
Kanto, Japan[24]	Witnessed OHCA (4068)	30-day survival with favorable neuro outcome	27/439 (6%) vs 30/712 (4%) 1.46 [0.88–2.42]
Osaka, Japan[25]	Witnessed OHCA of presumed cardiac origin (4902)	1-year survival with favorable neuro outcome	19/544 (3.5%) vs 28/783 (3.6%) 0.98 [0.55–1.73]
Sweden[26]	All OHCA with bystander CPR (11,275)	1-month survival	77/1145 (6.7%) vs 591/8209 (7.2%) 0.93 [0.74–1.17]
Norway[27]	All OHCA (695)	Survival to hospital discharge	15/145 (10%) vs 35/281 (13%) 0.83 [0.47–1.47]
Singapore[28]	All OHCA (2173)	Survival to hospital discharge	4/154 (2.6%) vs 8/287 (2.8%) 0.93 [0.29–3.05]
Arizona, USA[29,b]	Al OHCA of presumed cardiac origin (4415)	Survival to hospital discharge	113/849 (13.3%) vs 52/666 (7.8%) 1.7 [1.25–2.33]

Abbreviations: CI, confidence interval; RR, relative risk.
[a] RR and 95% CI calculated by authors of this review for ease of statistical comparison.
[b] Hands-only CPR taught as a recommended CPR technique.

plus rescue breathing (**Table 1**).[23–28] At the time of these studies, the only bystander CPR technique recommended or taught was chest compressions plus rescue breathing. Nevertheless, some bystanders chose to provide hands-only CPR without assisted ventilation, allowing for comparison of the two resuscitation strategies. Bystander CPR with or without rescue breathing substantially improved the rates of survival and survival with favorable neurologic outcomes compared with no bystander CPR.

In one of these studies the investigators evaluated 4068 witnessed cardiac arrests. Among the 1151 patients (28%) provided with bystander CPR, 439 (11%) received hands-only CPR and 712 (18%) received conventional chest compressions plus rescue breathing.[24] Six percent of these cardiac arrest victims survived with favorable neurologic outcomes at 30 days after hands-only CPR compared with 4% after conventional CPR (odds ratio [OR] 1.5; 95% confidence interval [CI], 0.9–2.5). Only 38% of the bystanders who provided hands-only CPR had prior CPR training versus 67% of the bystanders who provided conventional CPR. These data indicate that the cohort of bystanders who provided hands-only CPR were less well-trained than the cohort who provided conventional CPR, yet the outcomes were at least as good with hands-only CPR.

In 2010, Bobrow and colleagues[29] were the first to report outcomes from bystander hands-only CPR versus conventional CPR after a campaign to encourage bystanders to use hands-only CPR (ie, hands-only CPR was taught as a recommended CPR technique). The statewide multifaceted campaign in Arizona included online video training, in-person free hands-only CPR training (primarily sponsored by fire departments), school CPR training, public service announcements by the governor and local sports celebrities, and prominent publicity in

Table 2			
Clinical trials of telephone dispatcher-assisted CPR			
Location	Sample Size (N)	Primary End Point	Hands-Only CPR Vs Conventional CPR RR [95% CI][a]
Seattle[30]	520	Survival to hospital discharge	35/241 (14.6%) vs 29/279 (10.4%) 1.40 [0.88–2.22]
London, Washington (state)[31]	1941	Survival to hospital discharge	122/978 (12.5%) vs 105/956 (11.0%) 1.13 [0.89–1.45]
Sweden[32]	1276	30-day survival	54/620 (8.7%) vs 46/656 (7.0%) 1.24 [0.85–1.81]
NA (metaanalysis)[33]	3031	Survival to hospital discharge	211/1500 (14%) vs 178/1531 (12%) 1.21 [1.01–1.46]

Abbreviations: CI, confidence interval; NA, not applicable; RR, relative risk.
[a] RR and 95% CI calculated by authors of this review for ease of statistical comparison.

newspapers and television. The effort improved the bystander CPR rate from 28% to 40% ($P<.001$), and the proportion of CPR that was hands-only CPR increased from 19.6% to 75.9% ($P<.001$). Impressively, survival to hospital discharge rate was 13.3% (113 of 849) with hands-only bystander CPR versus 7.7% (52 of 666) with conventional CPR (adjusted OR 1.60; 95% CI, 1.08–2.35). Although these results are remarkable and underscore the potential benefit of widespread adoption of hands-only CPR, this study is inherently limited by the usual potential sources of bias associated with a prospective observational cohort design. The gold standard is a randomized controlled trial, but such a trial for bystander CPR is a daunting task.

Telephone Dispatcher-Assisted CPR

One opportunity for randomized controlled trials of bystander CPR is in the setting of telephone dispatcher-assisted CPR. In the 1990s, Hallstrom and colleagues[30] compared hands-only dispatcher-assisted bystander CPR with dispatcher-assisted conventional chest compressions plus rescue breathing. The investigators found that 14.6% survived to hospital discharge in the hands-only group versus 10.4% in the conventional group ($P = .18$). Although the results fell short of statistical significance, they suggested a potentially clinically important difference. Therefore, this issue was reexamined in two separate randomized controlled trials published in 2010; one conducted in the state of Washington and London[31] and another in Sweden.[32] Once again, both studies showed no statistically significant differences in outcomes, but the trends seemed to favor hands-only CPR (**Table 2**).

A metaanalysis of these three telephone dispatcher-assisted controlled trials revealed that hands-only CPR was associated with improved chance of survival-to-hospital discharge compared with conventional CPR (14% [211 of 1500] vs 12% [178 of 1531]; risk ratio 1.22, 95% CI 1.01–1.46).[33] Based on these studies, hands-only CPR is the recommended approach for telephone dispatcher-assisted CPR. It should be noted that the superior outcomes could be attributed in part to the difficulty of teaching mouth-to-mouth rescue breathing by telephone.

WHAT IS THE DOWNSIDE OF HANDS-ONLY CPR?
Is Assisted Ventilation Important for Asphyxial Cardiac Arrests in Animals?

Animal studies of CPR for cardiac arrests caused by acute asphyxia (asphyxial cardiac arrests) have established that assisted ventilation is an important component of CPR for asphyxial cardiac arrests.[34–36] In swine with acute asphyxial cardiac arrests after endotracheal tube clamping, the combination of chest compressions plus assisted ventilation improved systemic oxygenation, coronary perfusion pressures, early return of spontaneous circulation, and 24-hour survival compared with hands-only CPR.[34] In a similar study, piglets were provided with hands-only CPR versus conventional CPR with assisted ventilation versus no CPR for 8 minutes of simulated bystander CPR after endotracheal tube clamping until the systolic arterial pressure was greater than 50 mmHg. This model was intended to simulate bystander CPR for a pulseless patient who had sustained an acute asphyxial event such as a drowning episode. The best outcomes were in the group treated with chest compressions plus assisted ventilation; however, hands-only CPR also resulted in superior arterial and mixed venous blood gases and higher rates of 24-hour survival compared with no bystander CPR.[35]

Why Is Assisted Ventilation Important for an Asphyxial Cardiac Arrest?

During asphyxia, oxygen consumption, carbon dioxide production, and lactate production continue for many minutes before severe hypotension (pulselessness) or cardiac arrest. Peripheral and pulmonary blood flow continues prior to cardiac arrest, depleting the prearrest pulmonary oxygen reservoir. Thus, at the onset of CPR, there is substantial arterial hypoxemia, tissue hypoxia, and acidosis. Not surprising, assisted ventilation can be lifesaving in this setting.

Observational Studies Against Hands-Only Bystander CPR

Prolonged bystander CPR period

Consistent with the concerns raised in animal investigations, several observational studies indicate that rescue breathing is critically important in some circumstances, especially for prolonged CPR and for asphyxial cardiac arrests (**Table 3**). In a large Japanese study, Iwami and colleagues[25] showed that bystander hands-only CPR and conventional CPR were similarly effective for most adult OHCA. However, an a priori determined subgroup analysis revealed that conventional CPR was associated with better 1-year survival with favorable neurologic outcome than hands-only CPR among patients with a prolonged bystander CPR period of greater than 15 minutes from collapse to emergency medical services (EMS) resuscitation (2.2% [2 of 264] vs 0% [0 of 92], P<.05).[25] Kitamura and colleagues[37] reevaluated the question of resuscitation approach among victims with greater than 15 minutes from collapse to EMS resuscitation among more than 55,000 witnessed OHCAs during a 3-year period in the All-Japan Utstein Registry.[37] They showed that conventional bystander CPR resulted in a significantly higher rate of survival with favorable neurologic outcome compared with hands-only bystander CPR (2.0% [55 of 2707] vs 1.3% [36 of 2846], adjusted OR, 1.56; 95% CI, 1.02–2.44). Although statistically significant, the absolute survival is low regardless of type of CPR among this group. Even among the more than 55,000 witnessed OHCAs over 3 years in an entire large country, more than 20 additional patients with a prolonged bystander CPR period survived with a favorable neurologic outcome following conventional CPR compared with hands-only CPR.

Cardiac arrests from noncardiac causes

Because animal data and physiological concepts reviewed previously indicate that assisted ventilation is important for asphyxial cardiac arrests, Kitamura and colleagues[38] compared outcomes after hands-only bystander CPR versus conventional bystander CPR versus no bystander CPR among 43,246 bystander-witnessed , the conventional CPR group had a higher rate of survival with favorable neurologic

Table 3
Observational studies or subgroup analyses of bystander CPR in OHCA: special circumstances when hands-only CPR is inferior to conventional CPR

Location	Population or Subgroup (N)	Primary End Point	Hands-Only CPR Vs Conventional CPR RR [95% CI][a]
Osaka, Japan[25]	Long-duration cardiac arrests (>15 min) (864)	1-year survival with favorable neuro outcome	0/92 (0%) vs 3/139 (2.2%) 0 [0.00–undefined]
Japan[37]	Long-duration cardiac arrests (>15 min) of cardiac origin (11,704)	1-month survival with favorable neuro outcome	36/2846 (1.3%) vs 55/2707 (2.0%) 0.62 [0.41–0.94]
Japan[38]	OHCA of noncardiac origin (43,246)	1-month survival with favorable neuro outcome	131/8878 (1.5%) vs 136/7474 (1.8%) 0.81 [0.64–1.03]
Japan[39]	Pediatric OHCA of noncardiac origin (2297)	1-month survival with favorable neuro outcome	6/380 (1.6%) vs 45/624 (7.2%) 0.22 [0.09–0.51]
Japan[39]	Pediatric OHCA of cardiac origin (779)	1-month survival with favorable neuro outcome	14/158 (8.9%) vs 28/282 (9.9%) 0.89 [0.48–164]

Abbreviations: CI, confidence interval; RR, relative risk.
[a] RR and 95% CI calculated by authors of this review for ease of statistical comparison.

outcome 1 month postarrest (1.8%) than either the compression-only CPR group (1.5%; OR, 1.32; 95% CI, 1.03–1.69) or the no CPR group (1.4%; OR, 1.58; 95% CI, 1.28–1.96). Notably, this study indicates that rescue breathing has an incremental benefit for OHCAs of noncardiac origin, but the impact on the overall survival after OHCA was small due to the generally poor outcomes seen in OHCAs of noncardiac origin. Specifically, the number of OHCAs needed to treat with conventional CPR versus compression-only CPR to save a life with favorable neurologic outcome after OHCA was 290.

Unlike adult OHCAs, which are mostly from cardiac origins, pediatric OHCAs are mostly from noncardiac origin. Among 5170 children with OHCAs in the All-Japan Utstein Registry, 3675 (71%) had arrests of noncardiac causes and 1495 (29%) of cardiac causes.[39] Overall, favorable neurologic outcome was more common after conventional bystander CPR compared with hands-only CPR (7.2% [45of 624] vs 1.6% [6 of 380]; OR 5.54, 95% CI 2.52–16.99). Among children with OHCAs of cardiac cause, the rate of favorable neurologic outcome was not different between the conventional and hands-only bystander CPR groups (9.9% [28 of 282] vs 8.9% [14 of 158]; OR 1.20, 95% CI 0.55–2.66). Importantly, the rate of favorable neurologic outcome was more common after bystander CPR than no CPR (9.5% [42 of 440] vs 4.1% [14 of 339]; OR 2.21, 95% CI 1.08–4.54). These pediatric OHCA data are consistent with the adult data supporting hands-only CPR for OHCAs of cardiac causes but not for OHCAs of noncardiac causes. Because most pediatric OHCAs are from noncardiac causes, the American Heart Association recommends bystander CPR with assisted ventilation for children.

IHCAs in adults and children are also most commonly attributed to acute asphyxia.[40] Only 25% of IHCAs in adults have a first documented rhythm of VF or ventricular tachycardia.[41] Therefore, it seems reasonable to continue to recommend conventional CPR (CAB or chest Compression plus Airway management and rescue Breathing) for most IHCAs.

Another publication from the All-Japan Utstein Registry reported worse outcomes after hands-only CPR compared with conventional bystander CPR for all OHCAs and seemed to refute the conclusion of previous studies.[42] However, the investigators were rereporting most of the same data noted previously from other All-Japan Registry studies with the subtle wrinkle of combining the adult and pediatric data. Again, they showed no differences after hands-only versus conventional CPR for adults or for children with OHCAs of cardiac causes but worse outcomes for children with OHCAs of noncardiac causes (ie, the same results as the previous studies). Notably, the published data in all of these Japanese studies included in this review were obtained at a time before hands-only CPR was taught or recommended. Future studies from Japan and other areas may differ because hands-only bystander CPR and hands-only telephone dispatcher-assisted CPR are increasingly taught in Japan and many other areas.

IS RESCUE BREATHING NECESSARY FOR CPR BY EMS PROVIDERS?

In 2003, data from Tucson, Arizona, showed that chest compressions were provided by EMS providers greater than 50% of the time that they attended patients in cardiac arrest, and that outcomes were dismal.[43,44] Further evaluation revealed that the protocols unintentionally directed much of the interruptions and delays in chest compressions (assessing airway, breathing and circulation, placing the automated external defibrillator pads, waiting for rhythm analysis, endotracheal intubation, and so forth). The resuscitation research team and the fire department worked together to develop a new protocol, cardiocerebral resuscitation, or minimally interrupted cardiac resuscitation, based on animal data and clinical observational data. This protocol included (1) 200 uninterrupted preshock chest compressions, (2) 200 uninterrupted postshock chest compressions before pulse check or rhythm analysis, (3) delayed endotracheal intubation for 3 cycles of 200 compressions and rhythm analysis, and (4) attempted intravenous or intraosseous epinephrine before or during the second cycle of chest compressions.[44,45] Passive oxygen insufflation with placement of an oral-pharyngeal airway and high-flow oxygen was recommended, but bag-mask ventilation at 8 breaths per minute was allowed. A modification of the protocol for

Table 4			
Observational studies of cardiocerebral resuscitation, or minimally interrupted cardiac resuscitation			
Location	Population (N)	Primary End Point	CCR/MICR Vs Conventional CPR RR [95% CI][a]
Wisconsin (rural)[47]	All OHCA (historical control) (181)	Neurologically intact survival	35/89 (39%) vs 14/92 (15%) 2.58 [1.50–4.47]
Arizona (urban)[45]	All OHCA (before-after training) (886)	Survival to hospital discharge	36/668 (5.4%) vs 4/218 (1.8%) 2.94 [1.06–8.16]
Kansas City, Missouri[48]	All OHCA of presumed cardiac origin (1436)	Survival to hospital discharge	47/339 (13.9%) vs 82/1097 (7.5%) 1.85 [1.32–2.60]

Abbreviations: CCR, cardiocerebral resuscitation; CI, confidence interval; MICR (minimally interrupted cardiac resuscitation; RR, relative risk.
[a] RR and 95% CI calculated by authors of this review for ease of statistical comparison.

adults with cardiac arrest of presumed cardiac cause was evaluated in Wisconsin with a before-after experimental design.[46,47] The modification was that the first EMS rescuer provided chest compressions and the second rescuer extended the patient's neck and then provided an oral-pharyngeal airway and oxygen by face mask (assisted ventilation was not provided). Survival to discharge and survival with favorable neurologic outcome increased from 20% and 15% to 47% and 39%, respectively, following implementation of the cardiocerebral resuscitation protocol.[46,47] Similar programs were initiated at other sites including the whole state of Arizona, with similar excellent outcomes (**Table 4**).[45,48]

Bobrow and colleagues[49] tried to delineate whether elimination of rescue breathing was an important component of this impressive improvement of outcomes from OHCAs in Arizona by comparing minimally interrupted cardiac resuscitation patients with no rescue breathing versus those with bag-mask rescue breathing. Among the 1019 adult OHCA patients in the analysis, 459 received passive ventilation and 560 received bag-valve-mask ventilation. Adjusted neurologically intact survival after witnessed VF/ventricular tachycardia OHCA was higher for passive ventilation (38.2% [39 of 102]) than bag-valve-mask ventilation (25.8% [31 of 120]; adjusted OR 2.5, 95% CI 1.3–4.6). Survival rates did not differ after passive ventilation and bag-valve-mask ventilation for unwitnessed VF/ventricular tachycardia and nonshockable rhythms.

SUMMARY

Increasing evidence supports the value of hands-only CPR. Hands-only CPR is a reasonable approach for a single rescuer providing CPR after a witnessed sudden collapse cardiac arrest. Furthermore, hands-only CPR is the treatment of choice for telephone dispatcher-assisted bystander CPR. However, rescue breathing should be added for OHCA with a prolonged bystander CPR period and for cardiac arrest of noncardiac cause in children and adults (mostly asphyxial). Because asphyxia is the most common cause of pediatric cardiac arrest, rescue breathing should generally be provided for pediatric cardiac arrest. Similarly, because asphyxia is the most common cause of adult IHCA, rescue breathing should generally be provided for adult IHCA.

REFERENCES

1. Travers AH, Rea TD, Bobrow BJ, et al. Part 4: CPR overview: 2010 American Heart Association Guidelines for Cardiopulmonary Resuscitation and Emergency Cardiovascular Care. Circulation 2010;122(18 Suppl 3):S676–84.
2. Nichol G, Thomas E, Callaway CW, et al. Regional variation in out-of-hospital cardiac arrest incidence and outcome. JAMA 2008;300(12):1423–31.
3. Berg RA, Hemphill R, Abella BS, et al. Part 5: adult basic life support: 2010 American Heart Association Guidelines for Cardiopulmonary Resuscitation and Emergency Cardiovascular Care. Circulation 2010;122(18 Suppl 3):S685–705.
4. Merchant RM, Yang L, Becker LB, et al. Incidence of treated cardiac arrest in hospitalized patients in the United States. Crit Care Med 2011;39(11):2401–6.
5. Kouwenhoven WB, Jude JR, Knickerbocker GG. Closed-chest cardiac massage. JAMA 1960;173:1064–7.
6. Chandra NC, Gruben KG, Tsitlik JE, et al. Observations of ventilation during resuscitation in a canine model. Circulation 1994;90(6):3070–5.
7. Berg RA, Kern KB, Sanders AB, et al. Bystander cardiopulmonary resuscitation. Is ventilation necessary? Circulation 1993;88(4 Pt 1):1907–15.
8. Noc M, Weil MH, Tang W, et al. Mechanical ventilation may not be essential for initial cardiopulmonary resuscitation. Chest 1995;108(3):821–7.

9. Berg RA, Wilcoxson D, Hilwig RW, et al. The need for ventilatory support during bystander CPR. Ann Emerg Med 1995;26(3):342–50.
10. Berg RA, Kern KB, Hilwig RW, et al. Assisted ventilation does not improve outcome in a porcine model of single-rescuer bystander cardiopulmonary resuscitation. Circulation 1997;95(6):1635–41.
11. Berg RA, Kern KB, Hilwig RW, Ewy GA. Assisted ventilation during 'bystander' CPR in a swine acute myocardial infarction model does not improve outcome. Circulation 1997;96(12):4364–71.
12. Kern KB, Hilwig RW, Berg RA, et al. Efficacy of chest compression-only BLS CPR in the presence of an occluded airway. Resuscitation 1998;39(3):179–88.
13. Ewy GA, Zuercher M, Hilwig RW, et al. Improved neurological outcome with continuous chest compressions compared with 30:2 compressions-to-ventilations cardiopulmonary resuscitation in a realistic swine model of out-of-hospital cardiac arrest. Circulation 2007;116(22):2525–30.
14. Assar D, Chamberlain D, Colquhoun M, et al. Randomised controlled trials of staged teaching for basic life support. 1. Skill acquisition at bronze stage. Resuscitation 2000;45(1):7–15.
15. Heidenreich JW, Sanders AB, Higdon TA, et al. Uninterrupted chest compression CPR is easier to perform and remember than standard CPR. Resuscitation 2004; 63(2):123–30.
16. Heidenreich JW, Higdon TA, Kern KB, et al. Single-rescuer cardiopulmonary resuscitation: 'two quick breaths'–an oxymoron. Resuscitation 2004;62(3):283–9.
17. Higdon TA, Heidenreich JW, Kern KB, et al. Single rescuer cardiopulmonary resuscitation: can anyone perform to the guidelines 2000 recommendations? Resuscitation 2006;71(1):34–9.
18. Kern KB, Hilwig RW, Berg RA, et al. Importance of continuous chest compressions during cardiopulmonary resuscitation: improved outcome during a simulated single lay-rescuer scenario. Circulation 2002;105(5):645–9.
19. Sanders AB, Kern KB, Berg RA, et al. Survival and neurologic outcome after cardiopulmonary resuscitation with four different chest compression-ventilation ratios. Ann Emerg Med 2002;40(6):553–62.
20. Bobrow BJ, Zuercher M, Ewy GA, et al. Gasping during cardiac arrest in humans is frequent and associated with improved survival. Circulation 2008;118(24):2550–4.
21. Clark JJ, Larsen MP, Culley LL, et al. Incidence of agonal respirations in sudden cardiac arrest. Ann Emerg Med 1992;21(12):1464–7.
22. Idris AH, Becker LB, Fuerst RS, et al. Effect of ventilation on resuscitation in an animal model of cardiac arrest. Circulation 1994;90(6):3063–9.
23. Bossaert L, Van Hoeyweghen R. Bystander cardiopulmonary resuscitation (CPR) in out-of-hospital cardiac arrest. The Cerebral Resuscitation Study Group. Resuscitation 1989;(17 Suppl):S55–69 [discussion: S199–206].
24. Cardiopulmonary resuscitation by bystanders with chest compression only (SOS-KANTO): an observational study. Lancet 2007;369(9565):920–6.
25. Iwami T, Kawamura T, Hiraide A, et al. Effectiveness of bystander-initiated cardiac-only resuscitation for patients with out-of-hospital cardiac arrest. Circulation 2007; 116(25):2900–7.
26. Bohm K, Rosenqvist M, Herlitz J, et al. Survival is similar after standard treatment and chest compression only in out-of-hospital bystander cardiopulmonary resuscitation. Circulation 2007;116(25):2908–12.
27. Olasveengen TM, Wik L, Steen PA. Standard basic life support vs. continuous chest compressions only in out-of-hospital cardiac arrest. Acta Anaesthesiol Scand 2008; 52(7):914–9.

28. Ong ME, Ng FS, Anushia P, et al. Comparison of chest compression only and standard cardiopulmonary resuscitation for out-of-hospital cardiac arrest in Singapore. Resuscitation 2008;78(2):119–26.

29. Bobrow BJ, Spaite DW, Berg RA, et al. Chest compression-only CPR by lay rescuers and survival from out-of-hospital cardiac arrest. JAMA 2010;304(13):1447–54.

30. Hallstrom A, Cobb L, Johnson E, et al. Cardiopulmonary resuscitation by chest compression alone or with mouth-to-mouth ventilation. N Engl J Med 2000;342(21):1546–53.

31. Rea TD, Fahrenbruch C, Culley L, et al. CPR with chest compression alone or with rescue breathing. N Engl J Med 2010;363(5):423–33.

32. Svensson L, Bohm K, Castren M, et al. Compression-only CPR or standard CPR in out-of-hospital cardiac arrest. N Engl J Med 2010;363(5):434–42.

33. Hupfl M, Selig HF, Nagele P. Chest-compression-only versus standard cardiopulmonary resuscitation: a meta analysis. Lancet 2010;376(9752):1552–7.

34. Berg RA, Hilwig RW, Kern KB, et al. Simulated mouth-to-mouth ventilation and chest compressions (bystander cardiopulmonary resuscitation) improves outcome in a swine model of prehospital pediatric asphyxial cardiac arrest. Crit Care Med 1999;27(9):1893–9.

35. Berg RA, Hilwig RW, Kern KB, et al. "Bystander" chest compressions and assisted ventilation independently improve outcome from piglet asphyxial pulseless "cardiac arrest". Circulation 2000;101(14):1743–8.

36. Botran M, Lopez-Herce J, Urbano J, et al. Chest compressions versus ventilation plus chest compressions: a randomized trial in a pediatric asphyxial cardiac arrest animal model. Intensive Care Med 2011;37(11):1873–80.

37. Kitamura T, Iwami T, Kawamura T, et al. Time-dependent effectiveness of chest compression-only and conventional cardiopulmonary resuscitation for out-of-hospital cardiac arrest of cardiac origin. Resuscitation 2011;82(1):3–9.

38. Kitamura T, Iwami T, Kawamura T, et al. Bystander-initiated rescue breathing for out-of-hospital cardiac arrests of noncardiac origin. Circulation 2010;122(3):293–9.

39. Kitamura T, Iwami T, Kawamura T, et al. Conventional and chest-compression-only cardiopulmonary resuscitation by bystanders for children who have out-of-hospital cardiac arrests: a prospective, nationwide, population-based cohort study. Lancet 2010;375(9723):1347–54.

40. Nadkarni VM, Larkin GL, Peberdy MA, et al. First documented rhythm and clinical outcome from in-hospital cardiac arrest among children and adults. JAMA 2006;295(1):50–7.

41. Meaney PA, Nadkarni VM, Kern KB, et al. Rhythms and outcomes of adult in-hospital cardiac arrest. Crit Care Med 2010;38(1):101–8.

42. Ogawa T, Akahane M, Koike S, et al. Outcomes of chest compression only CPR versus conventional CPR conducted by lay people in patients with out of hospital cardiopulmonary arrest witnessed by bystanders: nationwide population based observational study. BMJ 2011;342:c7106.

43. Valenzuela TD, Kern KB, Clark LL, et al. Interruptions of chest compressions during emergency medical systems resuscitation. Circulation 2005;112(9):1259–65.

44. Ewy GA. Cardiocerebral resuscitation: the new cardiopulmonary resuscitation. Circulation 2005;111(16):2134–42.

45. Bobrow BJ, Clark LL, Ewy GA, et al. Minimally interrupted cardiac resuscitation by emergency medical services for out-of-hospital cardiac arrest. JAMA 2008;299(10):1158–65.

46. Kellum MJ, Kennedy KW, Ewy GA. Cardiocerebral resuscitation improves survival of patients with out-of-hospital cardiac arrest. Am J Med 2006;119(4):335–40.

47. Kellum MJ, Kennedy KW, Barney R, et al. Cardiocerebral resuscitation improves neurologically intact survival of patients with out-of-hospital cardiac arrest. Ann Emerg Med 2008;52(3):244–52.

48. Garza AG, Gratton MC, Salomone JA, et al. Improved patient survival using a modified resuscitation protocol for out-of-hospital cardiac arrest. Circulation 2009;119(19): 2597–605.

49. Bobrow BJ, Ewy GA, Clark L, et al. Passive oxygen insufflation is superior to bag-valve-mask ventilation for witnessed ventricular fibrillation out-of-hospital cardiac arrest. Ann Emerg Med 2009;54(5):656–62,e651.

Mechanical Devices for Cardiopulmonary Resuscitation

Henry Halperin, MD, MA, FHRS

KEYWORDS
- Cardiopulmonary resuscitation • Mechanical devices
- Cardiac arrest • Critical care

The rhythmic application of force to the body of the patient is fundamental to the process of generating blood flow in cardiopulmonary resuscitation (CPR), but there is little agreement as to the optimal technique for applying that force. There is a great need for improved external chest compression techniques, because only an average of 5% to 15% of patients treated with standard CPR survive cardiac arrest,[1,2] and it is widely agreed that increasing the blood flow generated by chest compression will improve survival. Given the potential importance of newer devices and techniques that may augment blood flow, this article explores several alternate devices and techniques that have been studied.

PISTON CHEST COMPRESSION

According to the most recently published guidelines of the Emergency Cardiac Care Committee of the American Heart Association,[3] external chest compressions are applied by the rescuer, who places the hands over the victim's sternum. Force is applied straight down with the elbows locked and the shoulders in line with the hands. The goal is to displace the sternum at least 2 inches for an average-sized adult victim 100 times per minute, with compression maintained for 50% of each cycle. Unfortunately, compressions are often done incorrectly,[4,5] and incorrect chest compression can compromise survival.[6,7] One way of potentially improving the quality of chest compression is with automatic mechanical devices, which can potentially apply compression more consistently than manually. Another way of potentially improving the quality of chest compression is to use gauges that provide feedback to the rescuer on the depth and rate of compressions, allowing the rescuer to adjust the application of force to produce compressions that have the correct depth and rate.

One type of automatic mechanical device uses a pneumatic piston (**Fig. 1**) to administer external chest compressions at a specified rate, compression depth, and duty cycle (percentage of time compression is held during each cycle). The piston is

Johns Hopkins University, Blalock 524, 600 North Wolfe Street, Baltimore, MD 21287, USA
E-mail address: hhalper@jhmi.edu

Crit Care Clin 28 (2012) 167–187
doi:10.1016/j.ccc.2012.02.002
0749-0704/12/$ – see front matter © 2012 Published by Elsevier Inc.

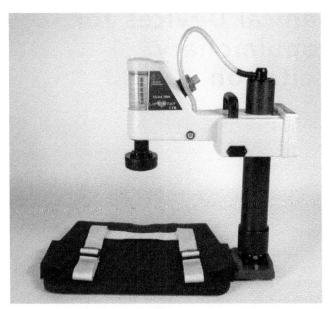

Fig. 1. Piston device used for performing mechanical external chest compressions. (Thumper, *Courtesy of* Michigan Instruments, Grand Rapids, MI.)

located at the end of an arm that extends over the patient's chest and is based on a board that provides a firm surface under the patient's back. In addition, a ventilation circuit is integrated into the device, which allows for continuous CPR with minimal operator input once the device is set up. Although there are some differences between mechanical and manual external chest compression in the time course of application of force, which may affect hemodynamics,[8,9] one small study showed no difference in survival using the two techniques.[9] Two additional small studies suggested a slight hemodynamic benefit to CPR performed by the pneumatic piston, one using end-tidal CO_2, as a surrogate measure for cardiac output[10] and the other showing a slight improvement in mean arterial pressure (25 vs 31 mm Hg), although no statistical analysis was provided.[9] An updated version of the piston compression device moves the piston with higher velocity and produces increased vascular pressures in an animal model compared with the earlier version.[11] Despite these slight differences in hemodynamics, chest compression performed by a pneumatic device probably has the same physiology as manual chest compression and is generally considered an extension of the standard technique.

Trauma is the major complication from piston CPR. The reported incidence of trauma as the result of piston CPR can be as high as 65%.[12,13] The most frequent thoracic injuries, occurring more than 20% of the time, include chest abrasions or contusions, defibrillator burns, sternal and rib fractures, gastric dilation, and pulmonary edema. Even properly executed CPR can lead to injury.

Despite the substantial amount of trauma, however, the detrimental effects of trauma are unclear, because most research on the incidence of CPR-related trauma has focused on nonsurvivors of CPR who might have died even if no trauma had occurred. Improvements in outcome may be achieved by external CPR techniques that improve blood flow, but such improvement has not been convincingly

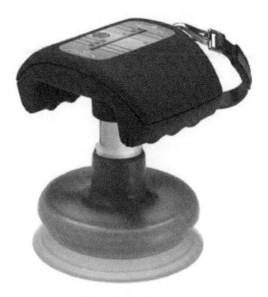

Fig. 2. Device for performing ACD-CPR. The upper part is a hand, whereas the lower part is a suction cup. (*Courtesy of* AMBU A/S, Denmark; with permission.)

demonstrated for piston-type devices. These devices do, however, allow CPR to be performed in situations where standard manual CPR would be difficult, such as in moving ambulances and where personnel are limited.

ACTIVE COMPRESSION-DECOMPRESSION CPR

In active compression-decompression (ACD), CPR is applied by using a compression device (either manual or mechanical) with an integral suction cup (**Fig. 2**). The suction cup allows for active decompression of the chest between compressions. Investigators studying this technique have used standard guidelines for the rate and duration of compressions. The decompression phase actively returns the chest wall to its expanded position without breaking contact. In human studies, ventilation has been performed according to the usual guidelines, but some animal studies have omitted ventilation except that caused by the compression-decompression itself.

ACD-CPR research began with a report of an elderly man resuscitated by his uninitiated son with a bathroom plunger.[14] Lurie and colleagues[14] at the University of California at San Francisco then began active research into the technique in both humans and an animal model. A device to perform ACD-CPR was developed by Ambu International (Copenhagen, Denmark), and numerous investigations have been performed with this technique.[15-35]

Physiology

ACD-CPR likely works in a fashion not dissimilar from interposed abdominal compression CPR, in which the active compression decompression serve to prime the intrathoracic pump mechanism.[36-39] The active compression decompression could result in greater chest expansion and filling with air between compressions, so that the next compression results in a greater rise in intrathoracic pressure and greater flow. A greater rise in intrathoracic pressure could be mediated through increased trapping of air in the lungs,[40] or simply increased application of force. Of note, chest compression force has not been measured in control groups undergoing standard manual CPR. Even if the peak compression forces used during active compression decompression CPR and standard CPR were comparable, it would still not be known whether the reported benefit for active compression decompression CPR results from the active compression decompression or from the increased force change (peak compression-to-peak decompression force) applied. For example, if 400 N compression force and 100 N decompression force were applied to the chest, is it equivalent simply to applying 500 N of compression force, or does the decompression force have unique physiologic effects that improve blood flow?

The active compression decompression could produce negative intrathoracic pressure between compressions and greater venous return, even without increasing the right atrial pressure relative to aortic pressure, which would impede coronary flow. Alternatively, there may be better right heart flow into the pulmonary bed between compressions. Additionally, the design of the device used for ACD-CPR results in the potential for a mechanism in the application of compression force that is slightly different from that in conventional CPR. In standard external chest compression the hands never lose contact with the thorax, and therefore the onset of application of force is gradual. The ACD-CPR device provides an air space of a few inches between the location of the hands and the chest wall. This gap allows some acceleration to take place before the force of compression actually reaches the chest, resulting in a slight impact on the chest wall. The significance of this impact with regard to the physiology of ACD-CPR is unknown. Studies reported to date have not resolved these issues. One study in pigs showed, in the absence of vasoconstrictors, increased coronary blood flow for active compression decompression CPR for a standardized amount of chest compression from a mechanical chest compressor.[41] Nevertheless, that same study showed no difference in coronary flow when vasoconstrictors were used.

A number of clinical trials have been reported with ACD-CPR. In the first clinical study, it was reported that 18 of 29 patients (62%) treated with active compression decompression CPR had return of spontaneous circulation (ROSC), compared with 10 of 33 patients (30%) treated with standard CPR. A number of larger clinical trials have been reported since that time. Most of the trials have shown no difference in survival for patients treated with standard CPR or ACD-CPR.[25,42–45]

In one trial in Paris, France, of 512 patients[30] there was an improvement in survival (ACD vs standard CPR) at 1 hour (36.6% vs 24.8%, $P = .003$, 24 hours (26% vs 13.6%, $P = .002$), and at hospital discharge (5.5% vs 1.9%, $P = .03$). Mean times from collapse to basic cardiac life support CPR was 9 minutes and from collapse to advanced cardiac life support CPR was 21 minutes. A later report of 750 patients from that latter group showed that survival was also improved at 1 year (5% vs 2%, $P = .03$).[32] All patients who survived to 1 year had cardiac arrests that were witnessed.

It is unclear why most trials showed no benefit for ACD-CPR over standard CPR and why there was a statistically significant, albeit small, benefit in Paris. It has been speculated that ACD-CPR may be of more benefit if administered relatively late in the course of cardiac arrest, as was done in Paris, and that the level of training and retraining is important.

There is a possibility that the high velocity of impact of the device at the start of chest compression could cause additional trauma as compared with conventional chest compressions.[46,47] In addition, the increased chest excursions produced by the active

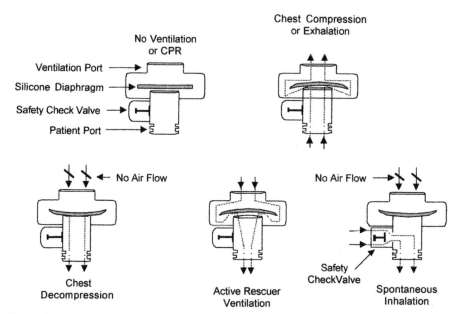

Fig. 3. Schematic of ITD. Components of the device are shown on the upper left panel. During chest compression or exhalation (*upper right panel*), air moves freely through the valve. During chest decompression (*lower left panel*), airflow is impeded by the device to increase the level of negative intrathoracic pressure generated. During rescuer ventilation or spontaneous inhalation (*lower middle and right panels*) air also moves freely through the valve. (*Adapted from* Lurie KG, Mulligan KA, McKnite S, et al. Optimizing standard cardiopulmonary resuscitation with an inspiratory impedance threshold valve. Chest 1998;113:1084–90.)

compression decompression could cause increased flexing of the ribs, and increased trauma.

Applicability

ACD-CPR shares the advantages of all manual techniques in that it is readily applied in a wide variety of circumstances. The device required to perform this technique could be made widely available should it prove significantly beneficial. The technique itself is not appreciably more difficult than standard external chest compression, although it may prove substantially more tiring, given that the rescuer is required to be active during both phases (compression and decompression) of each cycle.[48] The disadvantages of manual devices, however, are that an operator can perform the compressions incorrectly and chest compression must be interrupted for defibrillation.

IMPEDANCE THRESHOLD DEVICE

The impedance threshold device (ITD) is placed in the airway circuit to impede the flow of air into the chest during chest decompression (**Fig. 3**). Its goal is to increase the level of negative intrathoracic pressure generated during chest decompression, and thereby augment the beneficial effects of that negative intrathoracic pressure.

The ITD has been studied with standard CPR in a porcine model of cardiac arrest. In one study, coronary perfusion pressure (CPP) (diastolic aortic minus right atrial

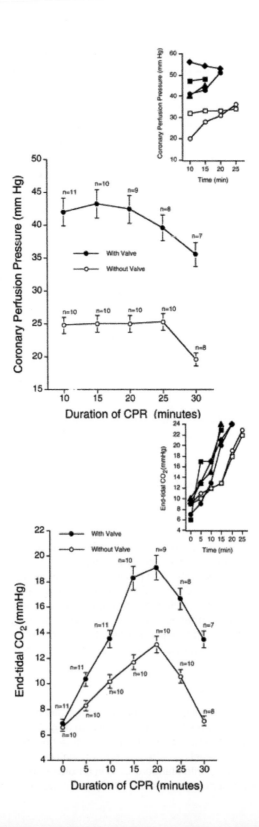

pressure) was the primary end point. After 2 minutes of CPR, mean +/− SEM CPP was 14 +/− 2 mm Hg with a sham valve versus 20 +/− 2 mm Hg in the ITD group (P<.006).[49] Significantly higher CPPs were maintained throughout the study when the ITD was used. In another study, microsphere-measured myocardiac blood flow was higher with the use of the ITD (0.32 +/− 0.04 vs 0.23 +/− 0.03 mL/min/g, P<.05), as was cerebral blood flow (0.23 +/− 0.02 vs 0.19 +/− 0.02; P<.05).[50] In a third study, the use of the ITD was evaluated to determine the potential to improve 24-hour survival and neurologic function in a pig model of cardiac arrest. The latter study used a randomized, prospective, and blinded design, where the effect of a sham versus active ITD was evaluated on 24-hour survival and neurologic function. After 6 minutes of ventricular fibrillation followed by 6 minutes of standard CPR with either a sham or an active valve, advanced life support was performed. A total of 11 of 20 pigs (55%) in the sham versus 17 of 20 (85%) in the active valve group survived for 24 hours (P<.05). Neurologic scores were significantly higher with the active valve; the cerebral performance score (1 = normal, 5 = brain death) was 2.2 +/− 0.2 with the sham ITD versus 1.4 +/− 0.2 with the active valve (P<.05).[51] Thus, with standard CPR in animal models, the ITD improved CPP, microsphere-determined myocardial and cerebral blood flows, and 24-hour survival and neurologic function.

Similar to the animal studies, clinical studies during manual cardiopulmonary resuscitation have shown a hemodynamic benefit for the ITD,[52] as well as improved short-term survival for patients with pulseless electrical activity with use of the ITD.[53] The ITD used with standard CPR has not, however, improved long-term survival in patients. In a recent large out-of-hospital study, patients receiving standard CPR had a fully functional (active) ITD or a nonfunctional (sham) ITD. Of 8718 patients included in the analysis, 4345 were randomly assigned to treatment with a sham ITD and 4373 to treatment with an active device. A total of 260 patients (6.0%) in the sham ITD group and 254 patients (5.8%) in the active ITD group had survival to hospital discharge with satisfactory neurologic outcome. There were also no significant differences in rates of ROSC on arrival at the emergency department, survival to hospital admission, and survival to hospital discharge.[54]

The ITD has also been studied in conjunction with ACD-CPR.[51,55,56] In a prospective, randomized, blinded trial performed in Paris, France, patients in nontraumatic cardiac arrest received ACD-CPR plus the valve or ACD-CPR alone for 30 minutes during advanced cardiac life support.[55] With the use of the ITD (**Fig. 4**) there were increases in end tidal carbon dioxide pressure (19.1 +/− 1.0 vs 13.1 +/− 0.9 mm Hg, P<.001), diastolic blood pressure (56.4 +/− 1.7 vs 36.5 +/− 1.5 mm Hg, P<.001), and CPP (43.3 +/− 1.6 vs 25.0 +/− 1.4 mm Hg, P<.001). In addition, ROSC was observed in 2 of 10 patients with ACD-CPR alone after 26.5 +/− 0.7 minutes versus 4 of 11 patients with ACD-CPR plus the ITD after 19.8 +/− 2.8 minutes (P<.05).

A prospective trial of ACD-CPR with the ITD versus standard CPR was performed in Mainz, Germany. Patients with out-of-hospital arrest of presumed cardiac pathogenesis were randomized to ACD+ITD CPR or standard CPR. The randomization was by rescuer crews, not individual patients. With ACD+ITD CPR (n = 103), ROSC and 1-hour and 24-hour survival rates were 55%, 51%, and 37% versus 37%, 32%, and

Fig. 4. CPPs (*left*), and end tidal CO_2 (*right*) in patients during ACD-CPR without (*lower tracing*) and with (*upper trancing*) the use of the ITD. (*From* Plaisance P, Lurie KG, Payen D. Inspiratory impedance during ACD-CPR: a randomized evaluation in patients in cardiac arrest. Circulation 2000;101:989–94; with permission.)

22% with standard CPR (n = 107) (P = .016, .006, and .033, respectively). One-hour and 24-hour survival rates in witnessed arrests were 55% and 41% with ACD+ITD CPR versus 33% and 23% in control subjects (P = .011 and .019), respectively. One-hour and 24-hour survival rates in patients with a witnessed arrest in ventricular fibrillation were 68% and 58% after ACD+ITD CPR versus 27% and 23% after standard CPR (P = .002 and .009), respectively. Hospital discharge rates were 18% after ACD+ITD CPR versus 13% in control subjects (P = .41). In witnessed arrests, overall neurologic function trended higher with ACD+ITD CPR versus control subjects (P = .07).[57]

A subsequent blinded, multicenter study was done to determine whether an inspiratory ITD, when used in combination with ACD-CPR, would improve survival rates in patients with out-of-hospital cardiac arrest. Patients were randomized to receive either a sham (n = 200) or an active ITD (n = 200) during advanced cardiac life support performed with ACD-CPR. The primary end point of this study was 24-hour survival. The 24-hour survival rates were 44 of 200 (22%) with the sham valve and 64 of 200 (32%) with the active valve (P = .02). The number of patients who had ROSC, intensive care unit admission, and hospital discharge rates was 77 (39%), 57 (29%), and 8 (4%) in the sham valve group versus 96 (48%) (P = .05), 79 (40%) (P = .02), and 10 (5%) (P = .6) in the active valve group.[58] Thus, whether the control group was standard CPR or ACD-CPR, the use of the ITD improved short-term survival.

In a recent study of out-of-hospital cardiac arrest, 2470 patients were provisionally enrolled and were randomly allocated to standard CPR or ACD-CPR with use of the ITD. Eight hundred thirteen (68%) of 1201 patients assigned to the standard CPR group (controls) and 840 (66%) of 1269 assigned to intervention CPR received designated CPR and were included in the final analyses. Forty-seven (6%) of 813 controls survived to hospital discharge with favorable neurologic function compared with 75 (9%) of 840 patients in the intervention group (odds ratio [OR] 1.58, 95% confidence interval [CI] 1.07–2.36; P = .019]. Seventy-four (9%) of 840 patients survived to 1 year in the intervention group compared with 48 (6%) of 813 controls (P = .03), with equivalent cognitive skills, disability ratings, and emotional-psychological statuses in both groups. The overall major adverse event rate did not differ between groups, but more patients had pulmonary edema in the intervention group (94 [11%] of 840) than did controls (62 [7%] of 813; P = .015).[59] A limitation of the latter study is the use of provisional enrollment.

Thus, the results with the ITD are promising. The device can be used with standard CPR as well as more advanced forms of CPR. There seems to be a hemodynamic benefit and short-term survival benefit with use of the device with standard CPR and a potential benefit in long-term survival with the use of the device with ACD-CPR.

LUND UNIVERSITY CARDIAC ARREST SYSTEM

The Lund University Cardiac Arrest System (LUCAS) piston technique was further modified by the addition of an integral suction cup (**Fig. 5**). The suction cup allows for active return of the chest to the neutral, uncompressed position and represents an evolution of the ACD technology. The current LUCAS device uses an electrically actuated piston for chest compression and decompression. In a series of 100 consecutive patients with witnessed cardiac arrest treated with the LUCAS device, if compressions were started less than 15 minutes after the ambulance call, the 30-day survival was 25% if the patients were in ventricular fibrillation, and 5% if they were in asystole.[60] If the device was placed more than 15 minutes after the ambulance call, there were no 30-day survivors. In a retrospective study of 508 patients in Sweden,

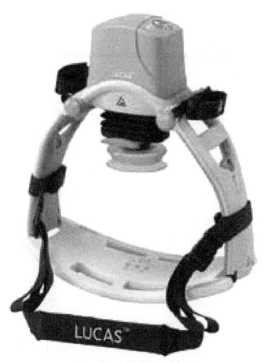

Fig. 5. LUCAS device (*Courtesy of* Physio-Control/Jolife AB, Lund, Sweden; with permission.). The device is positioned around the patient. The suction cup (at the lower end of the piston) adheres to the chest and is used to return the anterior chest to the neutral, uncompressed position in between chest compressions.

survival to discharge was assessed for patients treated with the LUCAS device as well as manual CPR.[61] A majority of the survivors had ROSC before application of the LUCAS device, making interpretation of that trial problematic.

To determine the extent of injuries that may be caused by the LUCAS device, an autopsy study was done comparing injuries from manual CPR with those from LUCAS CPR.[62] No injuries were found in 26 of 47 patients in the manual group and in 16 of 38 patients in the LUCAS group ($P = .28$). Sternal fracture was present in 10 of 47 in the manual group and 11 of 38 in the LUCAS group ($P = .46$), and there were multiple rib fractures ($>$ or $= 3$ fractures) in 13 of 47 in the manual group and in 17 of 38 in the LUCAS group ($P = .12$). It was concluded that injuries related to the use of the LUCAS device in this relatively small sample size were not different from those related to performing manual CPR.[62]

In preparation for a larger study comparing results from the use of the LUCAS device with those form manual CPR, a pilot study was performed.[63] Patients with out-of-hospital cardiac arrest were randomized to receive manual or LUCAS CPR. After exclusion, the LUCAS and the manual groups contained 75 and 73 patients, respectively. In the LUCAS and manual groups, spontaneous circulation with a palpable pulse returned in 30 and 23 patients ($P = .30$), spontaneous circulation with blood pressure above 80/50 mm Hg remained for at least 5 minutes in 23 and 19 patients ($P = .59$), the number of patients hospitalized alive greater than 4 hours were 18 and 15 ($P = .69$), and the number discharged, alive 6 and 7 ($P = .78$), respectively.

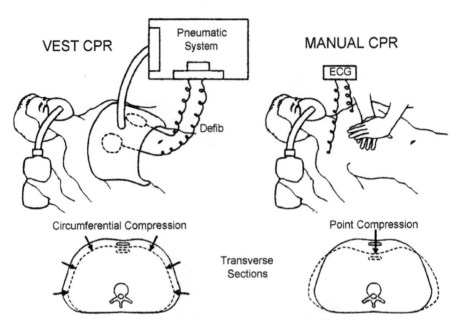

Fig. 6. Comparison of vest CPR and manual CPR. The vest is like a large blood pressure cuff that encircles the chest. A pneumatic system inflates and deflates the vest to compress and release the chest. Flat defibrillator (Defib) pads can be placed beneath the vest so that defibrillation can be performed during compressions. The vest compresses most of the circumference of the chest (*lower panels*), compared with a point compression of standard CPR. EGG, electrocardiogram. (*From* Halperin HR, Tsitlik JE, Gelfand M, et al. A preliminary study of cardiopulmonary resuscitation by circumferential compression of the chest with use of a pneumatic vest. N Engl J Med 1993;329:762–8; with permission. Copyright 1993, Massachusetts Medical Society.)

These data are being used to aid in the design of a larger clinical trial, including input for an appropriate power calculation.

VEST CARDIOPULMONARY RESUSCITATION

With vest CPR, a bladder-containing vest (analogous to a large blood pressure cuff) is placed circumferentially around the patient's chest (**Fig. 6**) and cyclically inflated and deflated by an automated pneumatic system. In this manner the chest is compressed cyclically. The device permits control of rate, compression duration, and inflation pressure. The vest also maintains a small amount of positive pressure on the chest between compressions to keep the vest snugly against the chest, except during the built-in pause for ventilation, at which time the vest completely deflates. The vest is generally inflated to a pressure of approximately 250 mm Hg, 60 times per minute, with 40% to 50% of each cycle in compression. Adherent defibrillation pads are placed on the chest before applying the vest to allow for defibrillation without having to remove the vest or interrupt CPR.

Vest CPR was developed as a means for augmenting intrathoracic pressure over that which could be produced by standard CPR. Vest CPR was largely developed by a group of investigators at Johns Hopkins University,[40,64–74] although other groups also made contributions.[75–84]

Physiology

Vest CPR is designed to maximize the intrathoracic pressure rises generated for a given force applied to the chest. By encircling the chest (see **Fig. 6**), force can be applied evenly, thus resulting in a large decrement in the volume of the chest with minimal displacement of an individual point on the chest wall. This circumferential compression allows for large increases in intrathoracic pressure without the trauma inherent in applying force to a single point, as with standard chest compression.

Many generations of vest CPR systems have been developed and tested. Studies with an early vest device reported by Luce and colleagues[83,84] in 1983 and 1984 showed that hemodynamics in a dog model of CPR were only minimally if at all improved with vest CPR compared with mechanically performed standard external chest compression. Niemann and colleagues[81] and Halperin and colleagues[64] used an improved system and showed augmentation of perfusion pressures and blood flows with vest CPR either with or without simultaneous ventilation. In the study by Halperin's group, survival was also better in the group of dogs receiving vest CPR. At high vest pressures they produced myocardial and brain blood flows equivalent to those in control animals, although they noted some trauma. At somewhat lower vest pressures, myocardial blood flow was 40% of prearrest flow, and cerebral blood flow was essentially equal to prearrest flow, with no trauma. These latter flows were greater than had been reported previously with standard external chest compression by any investigator.

Swenson and colleagues[75] reported a study of vest CPR in 10 patients late in cardiac arrest; they found no improvement in CPP produced with that vest CPR system. Halperin and colleagues[68] subsequently reported a two-phase study of vest CPR using an improved vest CPR system, which incorporated a vest that covered more of the chest than previous systems. This system also included a small positive pressure on the chest in between compressions to keep the vest tight against the chest. With the improved vest CPR system, hemodynamics in humans were significantly improved over those of standard external chest compression. Peak aortic pressure was nearly doubled (up to an average of 138 mm Hg), and CPP increased by 50%. A hemodynamic tracing during manual and vest CPR in a patient is shown in **Fig. 7**. In addition, 4 of the 29 patients had ROSC during vest CPR despite being late (50 ± 22 minutes) in resuscitation. The second phase of the study randomized patients to either vest CPR or standard external chest compression after initial (11 ± 4 minutes) advanced cardiac life support failed to resuscitate the patients. There was a trend toward improved initial resuscitation in the vest CPR group, but the trial was too small to show a statistically significant benefit.

If the vest is applied below the desired thoracic region, increased abdominal trauma could be expected. The vest does not, however, seem to increase the incidence of trauma over that of manual CPR,[68] although only limited data are available.

Applicability

Vest CPR requires a sophisticated device for its administration, which limits its use to locations where the device would be readily available. Application of the vest itself is not difficult and can be performed successfully by nurses, given only a few minutes instruction in its use. It is likely that if vest CPR proves successful in improving survival from cardiac arrest, it will remain predominantly in the hands of health care professionals. It will serve as a supplement, therefore, to the best form of standard CPR available for out-of-hospital arrests. Both animal and human data show rather

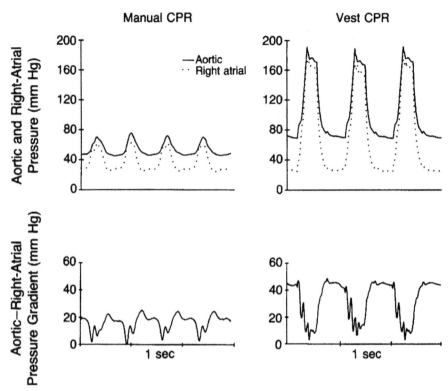

Fig. 7. Hemodynamic tracing during vest and manual CPR. Aortic, right atrial, and aortic minus right atrial pressures are shown. (*From* Halperin HR, Tsitlik JE, Gelfand M, et al. A preliminary study of cardiopulmonary resuscitation by circumferential compression of the chest with use of a pneumatic vest. N Engl J Med 1993;329:762–8; with permission. Copyright 1993, Massachusetts Medical Society.)

dramatic improvements in hemodynamics with vest CPR. If vest CPR can routinely raise the coronary perfusion gradient above the threshold required for late defibrillation to be successful, then it could make a measurable impact on the ability to achieve ROSC. Until sufficient human studies are done, however, we will not know whether or not this will result in improved long-term survival and neurologic recovery.

LOAD DISTRIBUTING BAND CPR

It had previously been shown that the circumferential vest device, analogous to a large blood pressure cuff that was inflated and deflated, could generate pressures during CPR that were substantially improved over those generated by standard CPR.[64,68] That vest device, however, was too large and consumed too much power to be easily portable and has not been tested in large clinical trials. An improved device, based on a band that distributes the compression load over the entire anterior chest (load distributing band; LDB) was subsequently developed.

Physiology

The LDB device probably has similar physiology to the vest CPR device, given that the compressive load is distributed over a large portion of the chest with both devices. An

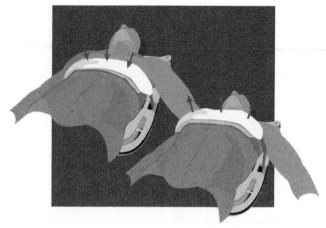

Fig. 8. Operation of the LDB device. During compression (*left*) the band is tightened by a motor and compression force is directed inward. During relaxation (*right*), the band is released and the chest expands.

initial animal trial showed that the LDB device generated peak aortic and CPPs that were improved over those generated with standard CPR.[85] An improved device was subsequently developed and was named the AutoPulse (**Fig. 8**). In a study using an improved LDB device, 30 pigs (16 ± 4 kg) were investigated comparing LDB-CPR with conventional CPR using the piston device (C-CPR). LDB-CPR improved CPP without epinephrine (LDB-CPR 21 ± 8 vs C-CPR 14 ± 6 mm Hg, mean ± SD, $P<.0001$) and with epinephrine (LDB-CPR 45 ± 11 vs C-CPR 17 ± 6 mm Hg, $P<.0001$). LDB-CPR improved myocardial flow without epinephrine and cerebral and myocardial flow with epinephrine ($P<.05$). LDB-CPR also produced greater myocardial flow at every CPP ($P<.01$). One of the mechanisms for the improved hemodynamics with LDB-CPR seems to be airway collapse (**Fig. 9**), trapping air in the lungs and resulting in higher and more sustained intrathoracic pressure generation not present with C-CPR.[86]

In a preliminary trial in terminally ill patients, following a minimum of 10 minutes of failed advanced life support, subjects received alternating periods of manual and LDB chest compressions for 90 seconds each. Peak aortic pressures were higher with LDB-CPR when compared with manual CPR (150 ± 8 vs 122 ± 11 mm Hg, $P<.05$, mean ± SEM), as was CPP (20 ± 3 vs 15 ± 3 mm Hg, $P<.02$), despite the fact that the manual chest compressions were of consistent high quality (51 ± 20 kg) and in all cases met or exceeded American Heart Association guidelines for depth of compression.[87] In that latter study, CPP was raised above the level generally associated with improved survival.[88]

In a case control study of LDB-CPR, a retrospective chart review was undertaken where a manual CPR comparison group was case-matched for age, gender, initial presenting electrocardiographic rhythm, and the number of doses of advanced cardiac life support medications as a proxy for treatment time. Matching was performed by an investigator blinded to outcome and treatment group. Sixty-nine LDB-CPR uses were matched to 93 manual CPR-only cases. LDB-CPR showed improvement in the primary outcome of survival to arrival at the emergency department when compared with manual CPR with any presenting rhythm (LDB-CPR 39%, manual 29%, $P = .003$). When patients were classified by first presenting rhythm, shockable

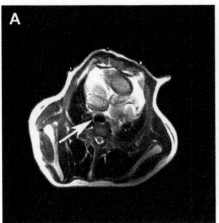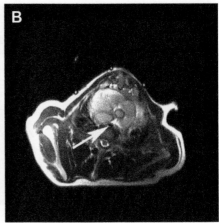

Fig. 9. Magnetic resonance imaging of the thorax during LDB-CPR in a pig. The trachea is widely patent in the uncompressed state (*A, arrow*) but is nearly fully collapsed during peak compression (*B, arrow*). (*From* Halperin HR, Paradis N, Ornato JP, et al. Cardiopulmonary resuscitation with a novel chest compression device in a porcine model of cardiac arrest: improved hemodynamics and mechanisms. J Am Coll Cardiol 2004;44:2214–20; with permission.)

rhythms showed no difference in outcome (LDB-CPR 44%, manual 50%, P = .340). Outcome was improved with LDB-CPR in initial presenting asystole and approached significance with pulseless electrical activity (PEA) (asystole: LDB-CPR 37%, manual 22%, P = .008; PEA: LDB-CPR 38%, manual 23%, P = .079).[89]

A prospective trial (ASPIRE trial) compared resuscitation outcomes following out-of-hospital cardiac arrest when an automated LDB-CPR device was added to standard emergency medical services (EMS) care with manual CPR. The trial included five centers and enrolled 1071 patients. Block randomization was done where a specific EMS crew would perform either LCD-CPR or manual CPR on a specific number of patients (block size), then perform the other type on a subsequent block of patients. In addition, the crews had the discretion of whether or not to enroll specific patients. The primary end point was survival to 4 hours after the 911 call. Following the first planned interim monitoring conducted by an independent data and safety monitoring board, study enrollment was terminated. No difference existed in the primary end point of survival to 4 hours between the manual CPR group and the LDB-CPR group overall (N = 1071; 30% vs 29%; P = .74). However, among the patients who were believed to have primary cardiac arrests, survival to hospital discharge was 9.9% in the manual CPR group and 5.8% in the LDB-CPR group (P = .06, adjusted for covariates and clustering). A cerebral performance category of 1 or 2 at hospital discharge was recorded in 7.5% of patients in the manual CPR group and in 3.1% of the LDB-CPR group (P = .006).[90]

There are a number of issues that make interpretation of the results of the ASPIRE trial problematic. A reanalysis of the data from the ASPIRE study showed that one site (Site C) made a potentially important protocol change midtrial, and enrollment at that site was noted to be independently associated with outcome.[91] The reanalysis was done post hoc, and all source data and documentation were considered using standard statistical approaches evaluating for possible secular, temporal, and trial design factors that may have related to the trial's outcome. The protocol change at Site C was found to have resulted in a delay in application of AutoPulse CPR. Before and after the protocol change, survival in patients receiving AutoPulse CPR decreased from 19.6% to 4% ($P = .024$). Logistic regression analysis showed Site C was significantly different ($P = .008$) from the remaining sites with respect to survival. Unlike Site C, the other sites actually showed an increase over time in the primary end point of 4-hour survival ($P = .008$) favorable to AutoPulse CPR. There did not seem to be significant safety ($P = .42$) or efficacy concerns ($P = .17$) at these sites. The survival with LDB-CPR and manual CPR were similar prior to the protocol change, but the survival with LDB-CPR decreased dramatically after the protocol change. The one statistically different site was responsible for the overall decrease in survival noted in the study. In addition to the change in protocol, other factors that could explain the decreased survival with LDB-CPR in the ASPIRE include (1) bias that could be introduced by the block randomization and crew enrollment discretion, (2) delays in performing defibrillation, and (3) inadequate training.[91]

A prospective and retrospective trial (Richmond trial) was conducted in Richmond, Virginia, comparing LDB-CPR with manual CPR after that EMS system switched from manual CPR to LDB-CPR. A total of 499 patients were included in the manual CPR phase (January 1, 2001, to March 31, 2003) and 284 patients in the LDB-CPR phase (December 20, 2003, to March 31, 2005); of these patients, the LDB device was applied in 210 patients. Patients in the manual CPR and LDB-CPR phases were comparable except for a faster response time interval (mean difference, 26 seconds) and more EMS-witnessed arrests (18.7% vs 12.6%) with LDB. Rates for ROSC and survival were increased with LDB-CPR compared with manual CPR (for ROSC, 34.5% vs 20.2%; and for survival to hospital discharge, 9.7%; 95% CI, 6.7%–13.8% vs 2.9%; 95% CI, 1.7%–4.8%; adjusted OR, 2.27; 95% CI, 1.11–4.77). In a secondary analysis of the 210 patients in whom the LDB device was applied, 38 patients (18.1%) survived to hospital admission (95% CI, 13.4%–23.9%) and 12 patients (5.7%) survived to hospital discharge (95% CI, 3.0%–9.3%).[92] A weakness of the Richmond trial was that there was a historical control group. A major strength was that all patients treated for cardiac arrest were included.

Applicability

Like vest CPR, LDB-CPR requires a sophisticated device for its administration, which limits its use to locations where the device would be readily available. The LDB device is, however, readily portable and can be applied in as little as 30 seconds. The LDB device will likely serve as a supplement, therefore, to the best form of standard CPR available for out-of-hospital arrests. Both animal and human data show rather dramatic improvements in hemodynamics with LDB-CPR, and there are mechanistic explanations for those improvements. If LDB-CPR can routinely raise the CPP above the threshold required for resuscitation, then it could make a measurable impact on the ability to achieve ROSC. LDB-CPR significantly improved survival in the Richmond trial, but not in the ASPIRE trial. The reasons that these two trials showed such differences in survival are unclear. There are likely implementation and training issues that have to be addressed. In addition, there is the fact that one site was responsible for the overall decrease in survival noted for the ASPIRE trial, likely due to that site's change in protocol midway through the trial. Another trial (CIRC) has just been completed that will address the issues noted in the previous trials and should be large enough to determine the true clinical utility of LDB-CPR.

THE FUTURE

Research aimed at improving survival from cardiac arrest both in-hospital and out-of-hospital continues. The first 45 years of external chest compression have been marked by enthusiasm, disappointment, innovation, and speculation, but to date no technique has convincingly positioned itself to replace standard CPR as we now know it. Research has contributed a great deal to the science of CPR and set the stage for real advancement in the resuscitation of cardiac arrest victims. The critical importance of early defibrillation is now clearly recognized, as is the importance of improved blood flow. Likewise, the criteria used to judge a new CPR method have been defined. These measures—CPP (important in predicting ROSC), systolic arterial pressure (predictive of cerebral blood flow and likely of neurologic recovery), and ultimately survival to hospital discharge—will drive the search for the best method or methods of applying force to the human body over the next several years. The future may lie not so much in a replacement of current CPR as in evolution to differing types of CPR under different circumstances, as well as improving the quality of standard CPR. Small hand-held devices are already under development that measure chest compression depth and compression rate to provide even lay rescuers with feedback to help them perform chest compressions at the specified 2 inches of displacement and 100 compressions per minute. Resuscitation initiated by lay persons will by necessity remain a manual technique, but some other form of CPR may be used once qualified rescuers are on the scene. Currently the distinction between basic and advanced life support involves the availability of drugs, mechanical airways, and defibrillation. It is very possible that the form of CPR used may also become part of this distinction, as well as the concomitant use of more advanced strategies such as hypothermia.

REFERENCES

1. Schneider AP 2nd, Nelson DJ, Brown DD. In-hospital cardiopulmonary resuscitation: a 30-year review. J Am Board Fam Pract 1993;6(2):91–101.
2. Tunstall-Pedoe H, Bailey L, Chamberlain DA, et al. Survey of 3765 cardiopulmonary resuscitations in British hospitals (the BRESUS Study): methods and overall results. BMJ 1992;304(6838):1347–51.
3. Berg RA, Hemphill R, Abella BS, et al. Part 5: adult basic life support: 2010 American Heart Association Guidelines for Cardiopulmonary Resuscitation and Emergency Cardiovascular Care. Circulation 2010;122(18 Suppl 3):S685–705.
4. Ochoa FJ, Ramalle-Gomara E, Lisa V, et al. The effect of rescuer fatigue on the quality of chest compressions. Resuscitation 1998;37(3):149–52.
5. Hightower D, Thomas SH, Stone CK, et al. Decay in quality of closed-chest compressions over time. Ann Emerg Med 1995;26(3):300–3.
6. Gallagher EJ, Lombardi G, Gennis P. Effectiveness of bystander cardiopulmonary resuscitation and survival following out-of-hospital cardiac arrest. JAMA 1995;274(24):1922–5.
7. Van Hoeyweghen RJ, Bossaert LL, Mullie A, et al. Quality and efficiency of bystander CPR. Belgian Cerebral Resuscitation Study Group. Resuscitation 1993;26(1):47–52.
8. Newton JR Jr, Glower DD, Wolfe JA, et al. A physiologic comparison of external cardiac massage techniques. J Thorac Cardiovasc Surg 1988;95(5):892–901.
9. McDonald JL. Systolic and mean arterial pressures during manual and mechanical CPR in humans. Ann Emerg Med 1982;11(6):292–5.
10. Ward KR, Menegazzi JJ, Zelenak RR, et al. A comparison of chest compressions between mechanical and manual CPR by monitoring end-tidal PCO2 during human cardiac arrest. Ann Emerg Med 1993;22(4):669–74.
11. Betz AE, Menegazzi JJ, Logue ES, et al. A randomized comparison of manual, mechanical and high-impulse chest compression in a porcine model of prolonged ventricular fibrillation. Resuscitation 2006;69:495–501.

12. Nagel EL, Fine EG, Krischer JP, et al. Complications of CPR. Crit Care Med 1981; 9(5):424.
13. Krischer JP, Fine EG, Davis JH, et al. Complications of cardiac resuscitation. Chest 1987;92(2):287–91.
14. Lurie KG, Lindo C, Chin J. CPR: the P stands for plumber's helper. JAMA 1990; 264(13):1661.
15. Sack JB, Gerber RS, Kesselbrenner MB. Active compression-decompression cardiopulmonary resuscitation. JAMA 1992;268(22):3200–1.
16. Cohen TJ, Goldner BG, Maccaro PC, et al. A comparison of active compression-decompression cardiopulmonary resuscitation with standard cardiopulmonary resuscitation for cardiac arrests occurring in the hospital. N Engl J Med 1993; 329(26):1918–21.
17. Tucker KJ, Khan JH, Savitt MA. Active compression-decompression resuscitation: effects on pulmonary ventilation. Resuscitation 1993;26(2):125–31.
18. Carli PA, De La Coussaye JE, Riou B, et al. Ventilatory effects of active compression-decompression in dogs. Ann Emerg Med 1994;24(5):890–4.
19. Chang MW, Coffeen P, Lurie KG, et al. Active compression-decompression CPR improves vital organ perfusion in a dog model of ventricular fibrillation. Chest 1994; 106(4):1250–9.
20. Sachs FL. Active compression-decompression cardiopulmonary resuscitation. N Engl J Med 1994;330(19):1391.
21. Wik L, Naess PA, llebekk A, et al. Simultaneous active compression-decompression and abdominal binding increase carotid blood flow additively during cardiopulmonary resuscitation (CPR) in pigs. Resuscitation 1994;28(1):55–64.
22. Schwab TM, Callaham ML, Madsen CD, et al. A randomized clinical trial of active compression-decompression CPR vs standard CPR in out-of-hospital cardiac arrest in two cities. JAMA 1995;273(16):1261–8.
23. Wenzel V, Fuerst RS, Idris AH, et al. Automatic mechanical device to standardize active compression-decompression CPR. Ann Emerg Med 1995;25(3):386–9.
24. Weston CF. Cardiopulmonary resuscitation with active compression-decompression. Br Heart J 1995;74(3):212–4.
25. Wik L, Mauer D, Robertson C. The first European pre-hospital active compression-decompression (ACD) cardiopulmonary resuscitation workshop: a report and a review of ACD-CPR. Resuscitation 1995;30(3):191–202.
26. Kern KB, Figge G, Hilwig RW, et al. Active compression-decompression versus standard cardiopulmonary resuscitation in a porcine model: no improvement in outcome. Am Heart J 1996;132(6):1156–62.
27. Malzer R, Zeiner A, Binder M, et al. Hemodynamic effects of active compression-decompression after prolonged CPR. Resuscitation 1996;31(3):243–53.
28. Schneider T, Wik L, Baubin M, et al. Active compression-decompression cardiopulmonary resuscitation–instructor and student manual for teaching and training. Part I: the workshop. Resuscitation 1996;32(3):203–6.
29. Baubin M, Schirmer M, Nogler M, et al. Active compression-decompression cardiopulmonary resuscitation in standing position over the patient: pros and cons of a new method. Resuscitation 1997;34(1):7–10.
30. Plaisance P, Adnet F, Vicaut E, et al. Benefit of active compression-decompression cardiopulmonary resuscitation as a prehospital advanced cardiac life support. A randomized multicenter study. Circulation 1997;95(4):955–61.
31. Mauer DK, Nolan J, Plaisance P, et al. Effect of active compression-decompression resuscitation (ACD-CPR) on survival: a combined analysis using individual patient data. Resuscitation 1999;41(3):249–56.

32. Plaisance P, Lurie KG, Vicaut E, et al. A comparison of standard cardiopulmonary resuscitation and active compression-decompression resuscitation for out-of-hospital cardiac arrest. French Active Compression-Decompression Cardiopulmonary Resuscitation Study Group. N Engl J Med 1999;341(8):569–75.

33. Steen S, Liao Q, Pierre L, et al. Evaluation of LUCAS, a new device for automatic mechanical compression and active decompression resuscitation. Resuscitation 2002;55(3):285–99.

34. Rubertsson S, Karlsten R. Increased cortical cerebral blood flow with LUCAS; a new device for mechanical chest compressions compared to standard external compressions during experimental cardiopulmonary resuscitation. Resuscitation 2005;65(3):357–63.

35. Babbs CF. Design of near-optimal waveforms for chest and abdominal compression and decompression in CPR using computer-simulated evolution. Resuscitation 2006; 08(2).277–93.

36. Lurie KG, Shultz JJ, Callaham ML, et al. Evaluation of active compression-decompression CPR in victims of out-of-hospital cardiac arrest. JAMA 1994; 271(18):1405–11.

37. Babbs CF. Circulatory adjuncts. Newer methods of cardiopulmonary resuscitation. Cardiol Clin 2002;20(1):37–59.

38. Babbs CF. CPR techniques that combine chest and abdominal compression and decompression: hemodynamic insights from a spreadsheet model. Circulation 1999; 100(21):2146–52.

39. Babbs CF, Thelander K. Theoretically optimal duty cycles for chest and abdominal compression during external cardiopulmonary resuscitation. Acad Emerg Med 1995; 2(8):698–707.

40. Halperin HR, Brower R, Weisfeldt ML, et al. Air trapping in the lungs during cardiopulmonary resuscitation in dogs. A mechanism for generating changes in intrathoracic pressure. Circ Res 1989;65(4):946–54.

41. Lindner KH, Pfenninger EG, Lurie KG, et al. Effects of active compression-decompression resuscitation on myocardial and cerebral blood flow in pigs. Circulation 1993;88(3):1254–63.

42. Nolan J, Smith G, Evans R, et al. The United Kingdom pre-hospital study of active compression-decompression resuscitation. Resuscitation 1998;37(2):119–25.

43. Panzer W, Bretthauer M, Klingler H, et al. ACD versus standard CPR in a prehospital setting. Resuscitation 1996;33(2):117–24.

44. Stiell IG, Hebert PC, Wells GA, et al. The Ontario trial of active compression-decompression cardiopulmonary resuscitation for in-hospital and prehospital cardiac arrest. JAMA 1996;275(18):1417–23.

45. Luiz T, Ellinger K, Denz C. Active compression-decompression cardiopulmonary resuscitation does not improve survival in patients with prehospital cardiac arrest in a physician-manned emergency medical system. J Cardiothorac Vasc Anesth 1996; 10(2):178–86.

46. Rabl W, Baubin M, Broinger G, et al. Serious complications from active compression-decompression cardiopulmonary resuscitation. Int J Legal Med 1996;109(2):84–9.

47. Baubin M, Rabl W, Pfeiffer KP, et al. Chest injuries after active compression-decompression cardiopulmonary resuscitation (ACD-CPR) in cadavers. Resuscitation 1999;43(1):9–15.

48. Shultz JJ, Mianulli MJ, Gisch TM, et al. Comparison of exertion required to perform standard and active compression-decompression cardiopulmonary resuscitation. Resuscitation 1995;29(1):23–31.

49. Lurie KG, Voelckel WG, Zielinski T, et al. Improving standard cardiopulmonary resuscitation with an inspiratory impedance threshold valve in a porcine model of cardiac arrest. Anesth Analg 2001;93(3):649–55.
50. Lurie KG, Mulligan KA, McKnite S, et al. Optimizing standard cardiopulmonary resuscitation with an inspiratory impedance threshold valve. Chest 1998;113(4): 1084–90.
51. Lurie KG, Zielinski T, McKnite S, et al. Use of an inspiratory impedance valve improves neurologically intact survival in a porcine model of ventricular fibrillation. Circulation 2002;105(1):124–9.
52. Pirrallo RG, Aufderheide TP, Provo TA, et al. Effect of an inspiratory impedance threshold device on hemodynamics during conventional manual cardiopulmonary resuscitation. Resuscitation 2005;66(1):13–20.
53. Aufderheide TP, Pirrallo RG, Provo TA, et al. Clinical evaluation of an inspiratory impedance threshold device during standard cardiopulmonary resuscitation in patients with out-of-hospital cardiac arrest. Crit Care Med 2005;33(4):734–40.
54. Aufderheide TP, Nichol G, Rea TD, et al. A trial of an impedance threshold device in out-of-hospital cardiac arrest. N Engl J Med 2011;365(9):798–806.
55. Plaisance P, Lurie KG, Payen D. Inspiratory impedance during active compression-decompression cardiopulmonary resuscitation: a randomized evaluation in patients in cardiac arrest. Circulation 2000;101(9):989–94.
56. Lurie K, Voelckel W, Plaisance P, et al. Use of an inspiratory impedance threshold valve during cardiopulmonary resuscitation: a progress report. Resuscitation 2000; 44(3):219–30.
57. Wolcke BB, Mauer DK, Schoefmann MF, et al. Comparison of standard cardiopulmonary resuscitation versus the combination of active compression-decompression cardiopulmonary resuscitation and an inspiratory impedance threshold device for out-of-hospital cardiac arrest. Circulation 2003;108(18):2201–5.
58. Plaisance P, Lurie KG, Vicaut E, et al. Evaluation of an impedance threshold device in patients receiving active compression-decompression cardiopulmonary resuscitation for out of hospital cardiac arrest. Resuscitation 2004;61(3):265–71.
59. Aufderheide TP, Frascone RJ, Wayne MA, et al. Standard cardiopulmonary resuscitation versus active compression-decompression cardiopulmonary resuscitation with augmentation of negative intrathoracic pressure for out-of-hospital cardiac arrest: a randomised trial. Lancet 2011;377(9762):301–11.
60. Steen S, Sjoberg T, Olsson P, et al. Treatment of out-of-hospital cardiac arrest with LUCAS, a new device for automatic mechanical compression and active decompression resuscitation. Resuscitation 2005;67(1):25–30.
61. Axelsson C, Axelsson AB, Svensson L, et al. Characteristics and outcome among patients suffering from out-of-hospital cardiac arrest with the emphasis on availability for intervention trials. Resuscitation 2007;75(3):460–8.
62. Smekal D, Johansson J, Huzevka T, et al. No difference in autopsy detected injuries in cardiac arrest patients treated with manual chest compressions compared with mechanical compressions with the LUCAS device–a pilot study. Resuscitation 2009; 80(10):1104–7.
63. Smekal D, Johansson J, Huzevka T, et al. A pilot study of mechanical chest compressions with the LUCAS device in cardiopulmonary resuscitation. Resuscitation 2011;82(6):702–6.
64. Halperin HR, Guerci AD, Chandra N, et al. Vest inflation without simultaneous ventilation during cardiac arrest in dogs: improved survival from prolonged cardiopulmonary resuscitation. Circulation 1986;74(6):1407–15.

65. Halperin HR, Tsitlik JE, Guerci AD, et al. Determinants of blood flow to vital organs during cardiopulmonary resuscitation in dogs. Circulation 1986;73(3):539–50.
66. Beattie C, Guerci AD, Hall T, et al. Mechanisms of blood flow during pneumatic vest cardiopulmonary resuscitation. J Appl Physiol 1991;70(1):454–65.
67. Eleff SM, Schleien CL, Koehler RC, et al. Brain bioenergetics during cardiopulmonary resuscitation in dogs. Anesthesiology 1992;76(1):77–84.
68. Halperin HR, Tsitlik JE, Gelfand M, et al. A preliminary study of cardiopulmonary resuscitation by circumferential compression of the chest with use of a pneumatic vest. N Engl J Med 1993;329(11):762–8.
69. Rudikoff MT, Maughan WL, Effron M, et al. Mechanisms of blood flow during cardiopulmonary resuscitation. Circulation 1980;61(2):345–52.
70. Weisfeldt ML, Chandra N. Physiology of cardiopulmonary resuscitation. Annu Rev Med 1981;32:435–42.
71. Weisfeldt ML. Recent advances in cardiopulmonary resuscitation. Jpn Circ J 1985; 49(1):13–24.
72. Weisfeldt ML, Halperin HR. Cardiopulmonary resuscitation: beyond cardiac massage. Circulation 1986;74(3):443–8.
73. Halperin HR, Weisfeldt ML. New approaches to CPR. Four hands, a plunger, or a vest. JAMA 1992;267(21):2940–1.
74. Weisfeldt ML. Challenges in cardiac arrest research. Ann Emerg Med 1993;22(1):4–5.
75. Swenson RD, Weaver WD, Niskanen RA, et al. Hemodynamics in humans during conventional and experimental methods of cardiopulmonary resuscitation. Circulation 1988;78(3):630–9.
76. Ben-Haim SA, Anuchnik CL, Dinnar U. A computer controller for vest cardiopulmonary resuscitation (CPR). IEEE Trans Biomed Eng 1988;35(5):413–6.
77. Ben-Haim SA, Shofti R, Ostrow B, et al. Effect of vest cardiopulmonary resuscitation rate on cardiac output and coronary blood flow. Crit Care Med 1989;17(8):768–71.
78. Raessler KL, Kern KB, Sanders AB, et al. Aortic and right atrial systolic pressures during cardiopulmonary resuscitation: a potential indicator of the mechanism of blood flow. Am Heart J 1988;115(5):1021–9.
79. Criley JM, Niemann JT, Rosborough JP, et al. Modifications of cardiopulmonary resuscitation based on the cough. Circulation 1986;74(6 Pt 2):IV42–50.
80. Criley JM. The thoracic pump provides a mechanism for coronary perfusion. Arch Intern Med 1995;155(11):1236.
81. Niemann JT, Rosborough JP, Niskanen RA, et al. Circulatory support during cardiac arrest using a pneumatic vest and abdominal binder with simultaneous high-pressure airway inflation. Ann Emerg Med 1984;13(9 Pt 2):767–70.
82. Niemann JT, Rosborough JP, Ung S, et al. Coronary perfusion pressure during experimental cardiopulmonary resuscitation. Ann Emerg Med 1982;11(3):127–31.
83. Luce JM, Ross BK, O'Quin RJ, et al. Regional blood flow during cardiopulmonary resuscitation in dogs using simultaneous and nonsimultaneous compression and ventilation. Circulation 1983;67(2):258–65.
84. Luce JM, Rizk NA, Niskanen RA. Regional blood flow during cardiopulmonary resuscitation in dogs. Crit Care Med 1984;12(10):874–8.
85. Halperin H, Berger R, Chandra N, et al. Cardiopulmonary resuscitation with a hydraulic-pneumatic band. Crit Care Med 2000;28(11 Suppl):N203–6.
86. Halperin HR, Paradis N, Ornato JP, et al. Cardiopulmonary resuscitation with a novel chest compression device in a porcine model of cardiac arrest: improved hemodynamics and mechanisms. J Am Coll Cardiol 2004;44(11):2214–20.

87. Timerman S, Cardoso LF, Ramires JA, et al. Improved hemodynamic performance with a novel chest compression device during treatment of in-hospital cardiac arrest. Resuscitation 2004;61(3):273–80.

88. Paradis NA, Martin GB, Rivers EP, et al. Coronary perfusion pressure and the return of spontaneous circulation in human cardiopulmonary resuscitation. JAMA 1990; 263(8):1106–13.

89. Casner M, Andersen D, Isaacs SM. The impact of a new CPR assist device on rate of return of spontaneous circulation in out-of-hospital cardiac arrest. Prehosp Emerg Care 2005;9(1):61–7.

90. Hallstrom A, Rea TD, Sayre MR, et al. Manual chest compression vs use of an automated chest compression device during resuscitation following out-of-hospital cardiac arrest: a randomized trial. JAMA 2006;295(22):2620–8.

91. Paradis NA, Young G, Lemeshow S, et al. Inhomogeneity and temporal effects in AutoPulse Assisted Prehospital International Resuscitation–an exception from consent trial terminated early. Am J Emerg Med 2010;28(4):391–8.

92. Ong ME, Ornato JP, Edwards DP, et al. Use of an automated, load-distributing band chest compression device for out-of-hospital cardiac arrest resuscitation. JAMA 2006;295(22):2629–37.

The Use of Vasopressor Agents During Cardiopulmonary Resuscitation

Kjetil Sunde, MD, PhD[a,b,*], Petter Andreas Steen, MD, PhD[a,c]

KEYWORDS
- Cardiac arrest • Cardiopulmonary resuscitation • Circulation
- Catecholamines • Vasopressin

Advanced cardiac life support (ACLS) during cardiac arrest combines cardiopulmonary resuscitation (CPR) with the use of a defibrillator, an advanced airway device, and drugs, most frequently vasopressors. The purpose of using a vasopressor during ACLS is not to increase cardiac output but to increase the perfusion pressure of the two most important and critical organs during CPR: the myocardium, for increased chance of return of spontaneous circulation (ROSC), and the brain, for increased chance of neurologically intact survival.

Coronary perfusion pressure (CoPP) is at any given time aortic pressure (AP) minus right atrial pressure (RAP) or myocardial tissue pressure (MTP), depending on which of the two is highest. With external chest compressions during cardiac arrest, RAP and/or MTP is usually as high as AP during compressions; thus, coronary perfusion only occurs during the decompression phase,[1,2] and only if decompression (diastolic) AP minus RAP is high enough. As expected, the level of CoPP above a certain threshold predicts ROSC and at least short-term survival both in animal and human cardiac arrest studies.[3,4]

Similarly, cerebral perfusion pressure (CePP) is at any time AP minus venous pressure or intracranial pressure (ICP), depending on which is highest. Cerebral perfusion differs from myocardial perfusion in that there is no stop in cerebral

This work was supported by grants from Health Region South East, Laerdal Foundation for Acute Medicine, and Anders Jahres Fund.
The authors have nothing to disclose.
[a] University of Oslo, PO Box 1171 Blindern, Oslo, Norway
[b] Department of Anesthesiology, Oslo University Hospital, PO Box 4956 Nydalen, N-0424, Oslo, Norway
[c] Prehospital Center, Oslo University Hospital, PO Box 4956 Nydalen, N-0424, Oslo, Norway
* Corresponding author. Department of Anesthesiology, Surgical ICU Ullevål, Oslo University Hospital, PO Box 4956 Nydalen, N-0424, Oslo, Norway.
E-mail address: kjetil.sunde@medisin.uio.no

perfusion during the compression phase (systole),[2,5] because myocardial contractions or chest compressions do not directly affect ICP. In fact, some animal studies indicate that cerebral perfusion is higher during the compression than the decompression phase.[5]

Various resuscitation techniques might therefore affect CoPP and CePP differently. Relative reductions in the duration of decompression often occurring with high compression rates might, for instance, reduce coronary perfusion but increase cardiac output and cerebral perfusion,[6] whereas an increase in AP without a concomitant increase in RAP will improve both coronary and cerebral perfusion if the resistance remains unchanged.

The latter is the rationale for using vasopressors, or more correctly, vasoconstrictors, during resuscitation. Drugs causing peripheral vasoconstriction with less effect on coronary or cerebral vascular resistance will shunt more of the cardiac output to these two critical organs. With increased peripheral resistance, cardiac output (and thereby end-tidal CO_2[7]) can in fact decrease while the perfusion of the heart and brain improves.[8,9] A decrease in end-tidal CO_2 after administration of a vasopressor[10,11] must therefore not be taken as a bad sign in itself.

CURRENT RECOMMENDATIONS

In adults, the 2010 American Heart Association (AHA) guidelines recommend administering 1 mg epinephrine intravenously (IV) or intraosseously (IO) every 3 to 5 minutes during ACLS, with 40 units vasopressin as an alternative for either the first or second dose.[12] No other drug is recommended as an alternative. For children, the recommended dose of epinephrine is 0.01 mg/kg IV/IO.[13] Vasopressin is not included in the pediatric algorithm, and the text states that there is insufficient evidence to make a recommendation for or against the routine use of vasopressin during cardiac arrest in children.[13]

Epinephrine has been an integral part of the CPR recommendations since the first standards were published in 1974.[14] Following is a closer look at the evidence behind these recommendations.

EPINEPHRINE, ANIMAL EXPERIMENTS

Animal experiments have shown increased CoPP when epinephrine is injected or continuously infused during CPR, with parallel increased macroscopic vital organ blood flow[15–17] and rate of ROSC.[18] The peripheral vasoconstriction with epinephrine is primary because of its α-adrenergic effects. However, recent studies have reported decreased microcirculatory cerebral blood flow with epinephrine given during CPR, which continued post-ROSC.[19,20] So, although increased macroscopic vital organ brain flow has been reported, the unwanted α_1-effects might decrease the microcirculatory vital organ blood flow at the cellular level.

Because epinephrine also has β-adrenergic effects, animal studies have indicated other potential harmful effects of epinephrine, including increased myocardial oxygen consumption,[21] postdefibrillation ventricular arrhythmias,[22] and increased post-ROSC myocardial dysfunction.[23] Angelos and colleagues[24] showed that with increased resuscitation duration, a paradoxical myocardial epinephrine response developed in rats, in which epinephrine was important to attain ROSC but with increasingly associated post-ROSC myocardial depression. Combining epinephrine with a β-blocker agent might therefore improve resuscibility and reduce post-ROSC myocardial dysfunction as indicated in other animal studies.[23,25] By blocking both the α_1 effects and the β_1 effects after epinephrine use, Pellis and colleagues[26] showed that the postresuscitation myocardial function was improved, with no differences in intraresuscitation hemodynamics. Further, the combination of epinephrine with glycerylnitrate[27] or a combination with epinephrine, vasopressin, and levosimedane[28] has shown promising results. Most recently, sodium nitroprusside during CPR improved outcome in a porcine cardiac arrest model.[29] Definitively, epinephrine alone does not seem to be the optimal choice, and more studies on drugs during CPR should be encouraged.

When a vasopressor is administered in a peripheral vein during ACLS, chest compressions are needed to circulate the drug. Pytte and colleagues[30] reported that in pigs, quality of CPR was important for whether peripheral vasoconstriction was achieved with epinephrine. The study was based on clinical prehospital data showing that chest compressions with a mean depth more shallow than guideline recommendations were given slightly less than half of the total ACLS time.[31] When pigs were given good quality continuous chest compressions, both CoPP and cerebral blood flow increased with increased femoral arterial resistance as expected, but with CPR quality equal to that found in the clinical studies, there was no effect of epinephrine on femoral resistance or coronary or cerebral hemodynamics.[30]

EPINEPHRINE, CLINICAL DATA

The fact that epinephrine has been a mainstay of ACLS for more than 40 years has not been based on good clinical data showing improved long-term survival. In fact, there have been no randomized controlled trials of epinephrine versus no epinephrine until very recently.[32]

In a study of 1391 patients before versus 4247 patients after introducing ACLS including IV epinephrine in ambulance services in Ontario, the rate of ROSC increased with ACLS, 10.9 versus 14.6 %, but with no increase in survival to hospital discharge, 5.0 versus 5.1 %.[33] In a similar study of 1296 patients, Ong and colleagues[34] found no improvement in ROSC rate or long-term survival after introducing epinephrine in an ambulance system, but the quality of that study was limited with rather poor protocol control.

Herlitz and colleagues[35] compared patients given epinephrine versus no epinephrine in a Swedish ambulance service in which only some personnel were authorized to give drugs. There was no difference in the frequency of hospitalization with ROSC, 36 % in both groups, but significantly fewer were discharged alive with epinephrine: 12 % of 417 patients versus 19 % of 786 patients.[35] In a large retrospective study of 10,966 patients (from the Swedish cardiac arrest registry) in which 42% of the patients received epinephrine, epinephrine was an independent predictor of a lower chance of survival (odds ratio 0.43) in a logistic regression analysis.[36] The regression analysis included factors such as place of arrest, witnessed/not witnessed, bystander CPR, presenting rhythm, age, and time from call to first CPR but not duration of CPR. Duration is a potentially important confounder because in many short resuscitation episodes, due to the success of the first defibrillation attempts the rescuers have not had time to administer any drug before ROSC.

Based on these data and speculating that a potential problem with epinephrine use might be inadequate CPR quality due to time for IV needle placement and drug administration, Olasveengen and colleagues[37] did a prospective, randomized study of IV needle placement and drugs versus no IV needle or drugs during out-of-hospital ACLS. Significantly more patients had ROSC and were hospitalized in the IV (n = 418) than the non-IV (n = 433) group (32 vs 21%) but with no difference in rate of survival to hospital discharge (10.5 vs 9.2%), good neurologic recovery (9.8 vs 8.1%), or 1-year survival (9.8 vs 8.3%).[37] The improvements in ROSC and hospital admission occurred in patients with initial nonshockable rhythms, with no difference for initial shockable patients. The individual contribution of epinephrine was not elucidated. The rather surprising finding in this study was that quality of CPR was very good in both groups with only median 14% versus 15% of the ACLS time without chest compressions in the non-IV group versus IV group, respectively.[37] It is discouraging that even with good quality CPR there was no significant improvement in long-term outcome with drugs, taking the findings of Pytte and colleagues[30] into consideration that good quality CPR might be required to obtain the wanted effects of epinephrine. This result indicates that we might not have the optimal drugs, or doses, in our current guidelines.[12,13]

It can be argued that an increased admission rate is positive with potential for better hospital treatment eventually causing better long-term survival. The great majority of in-hospital deaths were cerebral, however, and 71% to 72 % of patients in the two groups received therapeutic hypothermia,[37] the only brain-directed postresuscitation treatment at present. The other side of the coin is that the increased admission rate placed a heavy burden on the hospital intensive care units without more patients leaving the hospital alive, despite good quality postresuscitation care.[38] Still, it cannot be excluded that there is a type II statistical error with not enough patients entered into the study.

In a recent single-center double-blinded randomized study by Jacobs and colleagues,[32] epinephrine was compared with placebo in ACLS. As in the Olasveengen study,[37] the rate of ROSC increased with epinephrine (24% vs 8%), but with no significant difference in hospital discharge rate (4% vs 2%). Higher ROSC rates were found in both the shockable and nonshockable patients.[32] The study was planned with 5000 patients in five ambulance services, but four of the five decided not to participate for ethical reasons, so the study was underpowered for its primary end point of hospital discharge. Only 272 patients were recruited in the epinephrine group and 262 in the placebo group.[32]

EPINEPHRINE DOSE

So, although both studies indicate that epinephrine improves short-term survival, which dose is optimal? Animal experiments have indicated that 0.045 mg/kg gave better myocardial perfusion and ROSC rate compared with 0.015 mg/kg, 0.030 mg/kg, and 0.090 mg/kg (just statistically significant between 0.015 mg/kg and 0.045 mg/kg).[39] In a small clinical study by Paradis and colleagues, [40] high-dose epinephrine (0.2 mg/kg), increased CoPP more than the regular 1 mg dose, indicating an improvement in at least ROSC rate with high-dose epinephrine. This study was followed by several clinical studies of high-dose versus standard-dose epinephrine in adults. Woodhouse and colleagues[41] attempted to study high-dose epinephrine (10 mg) versus placebo in patients but ended with three groups: high-dose epinephrine, regular dose epinephrine, and placebo, because many participants violated the protocol and still gave 1 mg epinephrine. There was no difference between the groups in this poorly conducted study.[41] None of the other studies could show improved outcome with high-dose epinephrine, nor did a metaanalysis.[42] Pediatric studies are also consistent; no improvement with high-dose versus standard-dose epinephrine. There is even a trend toward lower survival with high-dose, significantly so in one study.[43] We might speculate that higher doses further improve resuscibility and ROSC rate but that all these short-term beneficial effects are lost because of the unwanted effects on cerebral microcirculation and postresuscitation myocardial dysfunction. This loss of benefit was recently shown in an experimental pig study[44] as in the previously mentioned study by Angelos and colleagues.[24] Thus, again, the search for alternatives to epinephrine is of utmost importance.

VASOPRESSIN, ANIMAL EXPERIMENTS

Arginine vasopressin, or antidiuretic hormone, is a peptide with strong nonadrenergic peripheral vasoconstrictive effects. It has been reported to cause cerebral vasodilatation[45] and both coronary vasoconstriction[46] and vasodilatation.[47] There are no unwanted direct β-adrenergic effects on the heart, and the effect duration is longer than for epinephrine.[48–50] The latter is an advantage during CPR but might cause a problem after ROSC if high afterload resulting from the vasoconstriction further increases the left ventricular myocardial dysfunction. In pig experiments, vasopressin increased survival with better neurologic outcome compared with epinephrine,[49,51] which was promising and led to several clinical studies.

VASOPRESSIN, CLINICAL DATA

Initial clinical studies with vasopressin were also promising.[52] Therefore, Wenzel and colleagues[53] performed a randomized multicenter study of vasopressin versus epinephrine during out-of-hospital cardiac arrest. There was no difference in rates of ROSC (24.6% vs 28.0%) or hospital discharge (9.9% in both groups) between 589 patients assigned to vasopressin and 597 to epinephrine, respectively.[53] Post hoc subgroup analysis showed better survival with vasopressin for patients with initial asystole (although with a high number of survivors with bad neurological outcome), but necessarily a trend toward the opposite for initial ventricular fibrillation or pulseless electrical activity because total survival in the whole study was identical.

In another clinical study from Canada, Stiell and colleagues[54] randomized 200 patients to vasopressin versus epinephrine in in-hospital cardiac arrest and found no significant difference in survival to hospital discharge, 12% versus 14%, respectively.

Aung and Htay[55] performed a systematic review and a metaanalysis of vasopressin versus epinephrine and found no difference in rates of ROSC, survival to hospital discharge, or survival with good neurologic recovery. They also failed to confirm an improvement with vasopressin for patients with initial asystole. Similar results have just been published in a metaanalysis by Mentzelopoulos and colleagues,[56] but they did describe that vasopressin may improve the long-term survival of asystolic patients, without, however, taking the neurologic outcome into account.[56]

Further post hoc analysis of the multicenter trial data indicated a positive effect of vasopressin combined with epinephrine versus epinephrine alone in patients with refractory cardiac arrest.[53] This result led to two randomized studies with a total of 4300 patients, with no improvement in rates of ROSC, long-term survival, or neurologic recovery for the combination of vasopressin and epinephrine versus epinephrine alone.[57,58] So, disappointingly, despite promising experimental data, vasopressin does not seem to improve outcome compared with epinephrine in cardiac-arrested patients.

OTHER VASOPRESSORS, CLINICAL STUDIES

Based on its unwanted effects with increased postresuscitation myocardial dysfunction[23,26] and reduced cerebral microcirculation,[19,20] epinephrine is unlikely to be the optimal vasopressor during ACLS. As stated before, the search for other vasopressors should be encouraged and further explored. In addition to vasopressin, norepinephrine, phenylephrine, and methoxamine have all been investigated in animals without showing any additional benefit to epinephrine. Some clinical studies have also been performed. Callaham and colleagues[59] compared high-dose (11 mg) and Lindner and colleagues[60] low-dose (1 mg) norepinephrine with 1 mg epinephrine. Although the rate of ROSC was higher, there was no improvement in survival to hospital discharge in either study.[59,60] Further, three randomized studies of variable doses of methoxamine versus epinephrine failed to find any significant improvement in rate of ROSC or survival.[61–63]

KNOWLEDGE GAPS

From the information cited previously, it seems clear that information is lacking on the optimal dose or timing of any vasopressor administration during ACLS. This conclusion is partly illustrated by differences in the 2010 European Resuscitation Council (ERC) and AHA guidelines. AHA recommends epinephrine administration after at least one shock and two minutes of CPR,[12] whereas ERC recommends it immediately after the third shock.[64] Does it matter if epinephrine is given just before, just after, or some time after a shock? Clinical data specifically addressing this question is lacking, but we know that it usually takes some time before a perfusing rhythm stabilizes postshock.[65] This time to stabilize is the reason for recommending continued chest compressions immediately after a defibrillation attempt without a rhythm check. In the authors' opinion, this scenario makes vasopressor administration just before or just after a shock questionable. If the shock results in ROSC, 1 mg of epinephrine is a very high dose for a myocardium that is just starting to contract again, most likely with dysfunction due to an acute myocardial infarction or the resuscitation procedure itself.[23] In addition, it takes time before a peripherally administered drug reaches its maximal vasoconstrictive effect. In pigs, CoPP peaked 70 to 90 seconds after peripheral drug administration with good quality chest compressions.[30] So, obviously, timing and pharmacokinetics will impact on drug efficacy during ACLS.

What about a continuous infusion versus traditional bolus administration? In a pig study, a bolus of epinephrine, 0.02 mg/kg, followed by a continuous infusion of 0.01 mg/kg/min increased cortical cerebral blood flow compared with repetitive doses of 0.02 mg/kg in pigs, but with no difference in jugular bulb oxygenation, CoPP, or ROSC rate.[17] Long-term survival and neurologic outcome, however, could have been affected, so this approach might deserve more attention.

SUMMARY

Epinephrine, both regular and high-dose, seems to increase the rate of ROSC during cardiac arrest treatment, but without improving long-term outcome. This result might be due to epinephrine's negative unwanted side effects like worsening of postresuscitation myocardial dysfunction and reduced cerebral microcirculation. It might also be due to lack of better brain-directed treatment beyond therapeutic hypothermia; we are able to bring more hearts back in patients in whom the brain is dead or dies. Vasopressin seems to be an acceptable alternative to epinephrine.

Laboratory data cannot be extrapolated to clinical CPR. There are possible species differences, most animals used are healthy with open coronary vessels, and factors influencing drug effects such as CPR quality and timing of drug administration are much better controlled in the laboratory. However, more research is needed in the treatment of cardiac arrest, both experimental and clinical, in the search for better drugs or combinations of drugs. Based on the current knowledge, the authors like to cite the latest ERC Guidelines[64]: "Although drugs and advanced airways are still included among ACLS interventions, they are of secondary importance to early defibrillation and high-quality, uninterrupted chest compressions."

REFERENCES

1. Kern KB, Hilwig R, Ewy GA. Retrograde coronary blood flow during cardiopulmonary resuscitation in swine: intracoronary Doppler evaluation. Am Heart J 1994;128: 490–9.
2. Steen S, Liao Q, Pierre L, et al. The critical importance of minimal delay between chest compressions and subsequent defibrillation: a haemodynamic explanation. Resuscitation 2003;58:249–58.
3. Kern KB, Ewy GA, Voorhees WD, et al. Myocardial perfusion pressure: a predictor of 24-hour survival during prolonged cardiac arrest in dogs. Resuscitation 1988; 16:241–50.
4. Paradis NA, Martin GB, Rivers EP, et al. Coronary perfusion pressure and the return of spontaneous circulation in human cardiopulmonary resuscitation. JAMA 1990;263: 1106–13.
5. Wik L, Naess PA, Ilebekk A, et al. Simultaneous active compression-decompression and abdominal binding increase carotid blood flow additively during cardiopulmonary resuscitation (CPR) in pigs. Resuscitation 1994;28:55–64.
6. Maier GW, Tyson GS Jr, Olsen CO, et al. The physiology of external cardiac massage: high-impulse cardiopulmonary resuscitation. Circulation 1984;70:86–101.
7. Gudipati CV, Weil MH, Bisera J, et al. Expired carbon dioxide: a noninvasive monitor of cardiopulmonary resuscitation. Circulation 1988;77:234–9.
8. Gonzalez ER, Ornato JP, Garnett AR, et al. Dose-dependent vasopressor response to epinephrine during CPR in human beings. Ann Emerg Med 1989;18:920–6.
9. Chase PB, Kern KB, Sanders AB, et al. Effects of graded doses of epinephrine on both noninvasive and invasive measures of myocardial perfusion and blood flow during cardiopulmonary resuscitation. Crit Care Med 1993;21:413–9.
10. Cantineau JP, Merckx P, Lamert Y, et al. Effect of epinephrine on end-tidal carbon dioxide pressure during prehospital cardiopulmonary resuscitation. Am J Emerg Med 1994;12:267–70.
11. Rubertsson S, Grenvik A, Zemgulis V, et al. Systemic perfusion pressure and blood flow before and after administration of epinephrine during experimental cardiopulmonary resuscitation. Crit Care Med 1995;23:1984–96.
12. Neumar RW, Otto CW, Link MS, et al. Part 8: adult advanced cardiovascular life support: 2010 American Heart Association Guidelines for Cardiopulmonary Resuscitation and Emergency Cardiovascular Care. Circulation 2010;122(18 Suppl 3):S729–67.
13. Kleinman ME, Chameides L, Schexnayder SM, et al. Part 14: pediatric advanced life support: 2010 American Heart Association Guidelines for Cardiopulmonary Resuscitation and Emergency Cardiovascular Care. Circulation 2010;122 (18 Suppl 3):S876–908.
14. Standards for cardiopulmonary resuscitation (CPR) and emergency cardiac care (ECC). 3. Advanced life support. JAMA 1974;227(Suppl):860–3.
15. Michael JR. Guerci AD, Koehler RC, et al. Mechanisms by which epinephrine augments cerebral and myocardial perfusion during cardiopulmonary resuscitation in dogs. Circulation 1984;69:822–35.
16. Lindner KH, Strohmengr HU, Prengel AU, et al. Hemodynamic and metabolic effects of epinephrine during cardiopulmonary resuscitation in a pig model. Crit Care Med 1992;20:1020–6.
17. Johansson J, Gedeborg R, Basu S, et al. Increased cortical cerebral blood flow by continuous infusion of adrenaline (epinephrine) during experimental cardiopulmonary resuscitation. Resuscitation 2003;57:299–307.

18. Brunette DD, Jameson SJ. Comparison of standard versus high-dose epinephrine in the resuscitation of cardiac arrest in dogs. Ann Emerg Med 1990;19:8–11.
19. Fries M, Weil MH, Chang YT, et al. Microcirculation during cardiac arrest and resuscitation. Crit Care Med 2006;34(Suppl):S454–7.
20. Ristagno G, Tang W, Huang L, et al. Epinephrine reduces cerebral perfusion during cardiopulmonary resuscitation. Crit Care Med 2009;37:1408–15.
21. Ditchey RV, Lindenfeld J. Failure of epinephrine to improve the balance between myocardial oxygen supply and demand during closed-chest resuscitation in dogs. Circulation 1988;78:382–9.
22. Niemann JT, Haynes KS, Garner D, et al. Postcountershock pulseless rhythms: response to CPR, artificial cardiac pacing, and adrenergic agonists. Ann Emerg Med 1986;15:112–20.
23. Tang W, Weil MH, Sun S, et al. Epinephrine increases the severity of postresuscitation myocardial dysfunction. Circulation 1995;92:3089–93.
24. Angelos MG, Butke RL, Panchal AR, et al. Cardiovascular response to epinephrine varies with increasing duration of cardiac arrest. Resuscitation 2008;77:101–10.
25. Ditchey RV, Rubio-Perez R, Slinker BK. Beta-adrenergic blockade reduces myocardial injury during experimental cardiopulmonary resuscitation. J Am Coll Cardiol 1994;24:804–12.
26. Pellis T, Weil MH, Tang W, et al. Evidence favoring the use of an alpha2-selective vasopressor agent for cardiopulmonary resuscitation. Circulation 2003;108:2716–21.
27. Kitsou V, Xanthos T, Stroumpoulis K, et al. Nitroglycerin and epinephrine improve coronary perfusion pressure in a porcine model of ventricular fibrillation arrest: a pilot study. J Emerg Med 2009;37:369–75.
28. Xanthos T, Bassiakou E, Koudouna E, et al. Combination pharmacotherapy in the treatment of experimental cardiac arrest. Am J Emerg Med 2009;27:651–9.
29. Yannopoulos D, Matsuura T, Schultz J, et al. Sodium nitroprusside enhanced cardiopulmonary resuscitation improves survival with good neurological function in a porcine model of prolonged cardiac arrest. Crit Care Med 2011;39:1269–74.
30. Pytte M, Kramer-Johansen J, Eilevstjønn J, et al. Haemodynamic effects of adrenaline (epinephrine) depend on chest compression quality during cardiopulmonary resuscitation in pigs. Resuscitation 2006;71:369–78.
31. Wik L, Kramer-Johansen J, Myklebust H, et al. Quality of cardiopulmonary resuscitation during out-of-hospital cardiac arrest. JAMA 2005;293:299–304.
32. Jacobs IG, Finn JC, Jelinek GA, et al. Effect of adrenaline on survival in out-of-hospital cardiac arrest: A randomised double-blind placebo-controlled trial. Resuscitation 2011;82:1138–43.
33. Stiell IG, Wells GA, Field B, et al. Advanced cardiac life support in out-of-hospital cardiac arrest. N Engl J Med 2004;351:647–56.
34. Ong ME, Tan EH, Ng FS, et al. Survival outcomes with the introduction of intravenous epinephrine in the management of out-of-hospital cardiac arrest. Ann Emerg Med 2007;50:635–42.
35. Herlitz J, Ekstrøm L, Wennerblom B, et al. Adrenaline in out-of-hospital ventricular fibrillation. Does it make any difference? Resuscitation 1995;29:195–201.
36. Holmberg M, Holmberg S, Herlitz J. Low chance of survival among patients requiring adrenaline (epinephrine) or intubation after out-of-hospital cardiac arrest in Sweden. Resuscitation 2002;4:37–45.
37. Olasveengen TM, Sunde K, Thowsen J, et al. Intravenous drug administration during out-of-hospital cardiac arrest: a randomized trial. JAMA 2009;302:2222–9.

38. Sunde K, Pytte M, Jacobsen D, et al. Implementation of a standardised treatment protocol for post resuscitation care after out-of-hospital cardiac arrest. Resuscitation 2007;73:29–39.

39. Lindner KH, Ahnefeld FW, Bowdler IM. Comparison of different doses of epinephrine on myocardial perfusion and resuscitation success during cardiopulmonary resuscitation in a pig model. Am J Emerg Med 1991;9:27–31.

40. Paradis NA, Martin GB, Rosenberg J, et al. The effect of standard- and high-dose epinephrine on coronary perfusion pressure during prolonged cardiopulmonary resuscitation. JAMA 1991;265:1139–44.

41. Woodhouse SP, Cox S, Boyd P, et al. High dose and standard dose adrenaline do not alter survival, compared with placebo, in cardiac arrest. Resuscitation 1995;30:243–9.

42. Vandycke C, Martens P. High dose versus standard dose epinephrine in cardiac arrest - a meta-analysis. Resuscitation 2000;45:161–6.

43. Perondi MB, Reis AG, Paiva EF, et al. A comparison of high-dose and standard-dose epinephrine in children with cardiac arrest. N Engl J Med 2004;350:1722–30.

44. Jeung KW, Ryu HH, Song KH, et al. Variable effects of high-dose adrenaline relative to standard-dose adrenaline on resuscitation outcomes according to cardiac arrest duration. Resuscitation 2011;82:932–6.

45. Suzuki Y, Satoh S, Oyama H, et al. Regional differences in the vasodilator response to vasopressin in canine cerebral arteries in vivo. Stroke 1993;24:1049–53.

46. Peters KG, Marcus ML, Harrison DG. Vasopressin and the mature coronary collateral circulation. Circulation 1989;79:1324–31.

47. Mayr VD, Wenzel V, Wagner-Berger HG, et al. Arginine vasopressin during sinus rhythm: effects on haemodynamic variables, left anterior descending coronary artery cross sectional area and cardiac index, before and after inhibition of NO-synthase, in pigs. Resuscitation 2007;74:366–71.

48. Wenzel V, Lindner KH, Prengel AW, et al. Vasopressin improves vital organ blood flow after prolonged cardiac arrest with postcountershock pulseless electrical activity in pigs. Crit Care Med 1999;27:486–92.

49. Wenzel V, Lindner KH, Krismer AC, et al. Repeated administration of vasopressin but not epinephrine maintains coronary perfusion pressure after early and late administration during prolonged cardiopulmonary resuscitation in pigs. Circulation 1999;99:1379–84.

50. Johansson, J, Gedeborg R, Rubertsson S. Vasopressin versus continuous adrenaline during experimental cardiopulmonary resuscitation. Resuscitation 2004;62:61–9.

51. Wenzel V, Lindner KH, Krismer AC, et al. Survival with full neurologic recovery and no cerebral pathology after prolonged cardiopulmonary resuscitation with vasopressin in pigs. J Am Coll Cardiol 2000;35:527–33.

52. Lindner KH, Dirks B, Strohmenger HU, et al. Randomised comparison of epinephrine and vasopressin in patients with out-of-hospital ventricular fibrillation. Lancet 1997;349:535–7.

53. Wenzel V, Krismer AC, Arntz HR, et al. A comparison of vasopressin and epinephrine for out-of-hospital cardiopulmonary resuscitation. N Engl J Med 2004;350:105–13.

54. Stiell IG, Hebert PC, Wells GA, et al. Vasopressin versus epinephrine for inhospital cardiac arrest: a randomised controlled trial. Lancet 2001;358:105–9.

55. Aung K. Htay T. Vasopressin for cardiac arrest: a systematic review and meta analysis. Arch Intern Med 2005;165:17–24.

56. Mentzelopoulos SD, Zakynthinos SG, Siempos I, et al. Vasopressin for cardiac arrest: meta-analysis of randomized controlled trials. Resuscitation 2011. [Epub ahead of print]. PMID: 2178773.

57. Callaway CW, Hostler D, Doshi AA, et al. Usefulness of vasopressin administered with epinephrine during out-of-hospital cardiac arrest. Am J Cardiol 2006;98:1316–21.
58. Gueugniaud PY, David JS, Channzy E, et al. Vasopressin and epinephrine vs. epinephrine alone in cardiopulmonary resuscitation. N Engl J Med 2008;359:21–30.
59. Callaham M, Madsen CD, Barton CW, et al. A randomized clinical trial of high-dose epinephrine and norepinephrine vs standard-dose epinephrine in prehospital cardiac arrest. JAMA 1992;268:2667–72.
60. Lindner KH, Ahnefeld FW, Grunert A. Epinephrine versus norepinephrine in prehospital ventricular fibrillation. Am J Cardiol 1991;67:427–8.
61. Olson DW, Thakur R, Stueven HA, et al. Randomized study of epinephrine versus methoxamine in prehospital ventricular fibrillation. Ann Emerg Med 1989;18:250–3.
62. Patrick WD, Freedman J, McEwen T, et al. A randomized, double-blind comparison of methoxamine and epinephrine in human cardiopulmonary arrest. Am J Respir Crit Care Med 1995;152:519–23.
63. Turner LM, Parsons M, Luetkemeyer RC, et al. A comparison of epinephrine and methoxamine for resuscitation from electromechanical dissociation in human beings. Ann Emerg Med 1988;17:443–9.
64. Deakin CD, Nolan JP, Soar J, et al. European Resuscitation Council Guidelines for Resuscitation 2010 Section 4. Adult advanced life support. Resuscitation 2010;81:1305–52.
65. Sunde K, Eftestøl T, Askenberg C, et al. Quality assessment of defribrillation and advanced life support using data from the medical control module of the defibrillator. Resuscitation 1999;41:237–47.

Optimizing the Timing of Defibrillation: The Role of Ventricular Fibrillation Waveform Analysis During Cardiopulmonary Resuscitation

Yongqin Li, PhD[a], Wanchun Tang, MD, Master CCM[a,b,*]

KEYWORDS

- Cardiac arrest • Cardiopulmonary resuscitation
- Timing of defibrillation • Ventricular fibrillation
- Waveform analysis

Despite important advances in prevention, cardiac arrest (CA) is still a leading cause of death in many parts of the world. The principles of cardiopulmonary resuscitation (CPR) have remained fundamentally unchanged during the past 40 years. Successful resuscitation is strongly associated with several specific interventions, including early bystander CPR,[1,2] earlier defibrillation, high quality of chest compressions,[3,4] and immediate postresuscitation care.[5]

Ventricular fibrillation (VF), which is characterized as rapid, disorganized contractions of the heart with complex electrocardiogram (ECG) patterns, remains the primary rhythm in many instances of CA. The only reliable method of treating VF is electrical defibrillation, which was first used in humans in 1947.[6] For every minute that passes between collapse and defibrillation, survival rates from witnessed VF decrease 7% to 10% if no CPR is provided. Even though earlier defibrillation during CPR is greatly emphasized, it is increasingly clear that not all patients in VF benefit from being treated in the same manner, as the duration of VF is a major determinant of countershock outcome.[7] If defibrillation is undertaken when the myocardial metabolic state is compromised, success rates are lower.[8,9] Repetitive high-energy defibrillation can also damage the already precarious myocardium.[9–11] For these reasons, the

[a] The Weil Institute of Critical Care Medicine, 35-100 Bob Hope Drive, Rancho Mirage, CA 92270, USA
[b] The Keck School of Medicine of the University of Southern California, Health Sciences Campus, Los Angeles, CA 90089, USA
* Corresponding author. The Weil Institute of Critical Care Medicine, 35-100 Bob Hope Drive, Rancho Mirage, CA 92270.
E-mail address: drsheart@aol.com

Crit Care Clin 28 (2012) 199–210
doi:10.1016/j.ccc.2011.10.013   criticalcare.theclinics.com
0749-0704/12/$ – see front matter © 2012 Elsevier Inc. All rights reserved.

ability to gain information concerning the metabolic state of the myocardium and to optimize the timing of defibrillation would be of enormous benefit in allowing therapy to be tailored to an individual heart.

IMPORTANCE OF OPTIMIZING THE TIMING OF DEFIBRILLATION

The major determinant of successful defibrillation is the duration of VF. There is evidence that when the interval between the onset of VF and the delivery of the first shock is less than 5 minutes, an immediate electrical shock may be successful.[12] However, both animal and human studies demonstrate that when the duration of untreated VF exceeds 5 minutes, initial CPR with chest compression before delivery of a defibrillation attempt improves the likelihood of restoration of spontaneous circulation (ROSC).[13,14] However, the duration of collapse may be difficult to access, especially in out-of-hospital patients. Analysis of the VF waveform may provide a measure of VF duration. However, more direct prognostic information that could be used to determine whether a patient should receive immediate attempted defibrillation or alternate therapy such as CPR or medications would be advantageous.

The evidence is clear that the quality of chest compressions is another major determinant of successful resuscitation. Successful shocks are associated with shorter preshock pause duration and higher mean chest compression depth in the 30 seconds preceding the preshock pause.[15] Established predictors of good-quality CPR therefore may be used to optimize the timing of defibrillation by predicting the success of defibrillation and thereby successful resuscitation.

On the other hand, more than 50% of patients initially resuscitated from CA subsequently die before leaving the hospital, and the majority of these deaths are due to impaired myocardial function.[16–18] The severity of postresuscitation myocardial dysfunction has been recognized to be related, in part, to the magnitude of the total electrical energy delivered with defibrillation.[19] Increases in the defibrillation energy are associated with decreased postresuscitation myocardial function.[19,20] Optimizing the timing of defibrillation therefore may decrease the severity of postresuscitation myocardial dysfunction by reducing the numbers of failed or unnecessary shocks.

The development of a noninvasive and real-time monitoring during CPR that provides substantial information to the rescuers and allows for optimizing the timing of defibrillation is of great importance to prioritize interventions, chest compression or defibrillation, to minimize the interruption in CPR, to reduce the number of failed defibrillation attempts, and ultimately improve the final outcome.

OPTIMIZING THE TIMING OF DEFIBRILLATION

The optimal timing of defibrillation is determined by evaluating the probability of shock outcomes. If the attempted shock has a high likelihood of defibrillation success, an electrical shock should be prompted and delivered. Otherwise, unnecessary shocks should be avoided and alternate therapy such as CPR or medications, especially high-quality chest compression, should be utilized. For the purpose of optimizing the timing of defibrillation, invasive hemodynamic measurements, especially coronary perfusion pressure (CPP)[21] and end-tidal CO_2 (EtCO$_2$), are employed.[22]

Experimentally, in a porcine model of CA and CPR, CPP and EtCO$_2$ above the threshold level of 15 mm Hg have been the only predictors of successful resuscitation, other than the priority interventions of chest compression or defibrillation.[22,23] Although the importance of CPP during CPR is clear, invasive measurements, including aortic and right atrial pressures, are available or feasible at the time of resuscitation in only a very small minority of patients in critical care settings. The use of EtCO$_2$ measurements is also not widely available, especially because of the need for endotracheal intubation.

Consideration, with the intent to identify a better predictor of defibrillation and ROSC, has therefore been focused on the analyses of electrocardiographic features of VF waveforms, which is routinely available in the current automated external defibrillators (AEDs).[24,25] The ECG recorded from the surface of the body represents the superposition of all of the electrical fields generated by each volume element of the heart.[26] Presumably, organization of the surface ECG has some relationship to the underlying organization of the myocardial electrical activity. VF waveforms change with time and exhibit predictable changes over time during CA and CPR (**Fig. 1**). VF waveform analysis therefore can be used to predict the probability of shock outcome, monitor the effectiveness of chest compression, optimize the timing of defibrillation, and ultimately guide CPR interventions.

OPTIMIZING THE TIMING OF DEFIBRILLATION BY VF WAVEFORM ANALYSIS

The search for defibrillation prediction features gained from VF waveforms dates back 20 years, and recently published review articles[24,26] provide excellent overviews of various techniques developed for VF waveform analysis and the resulting information

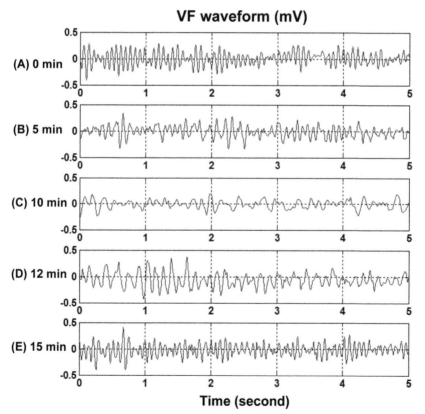

Fig. 1. ECG waveform recorded during untreated VF in a porcine model of cardiac arrest. (*A*) 0 minute of VF. (*B*) 5 minutes of VF. (*C*) 10 minutes of VF and CPR. (*D*) 12 minutes of VF. (*E*) 15 minutes of VF. CPR was initiated from 10 minutes of VF and lasted for 5 minutes.

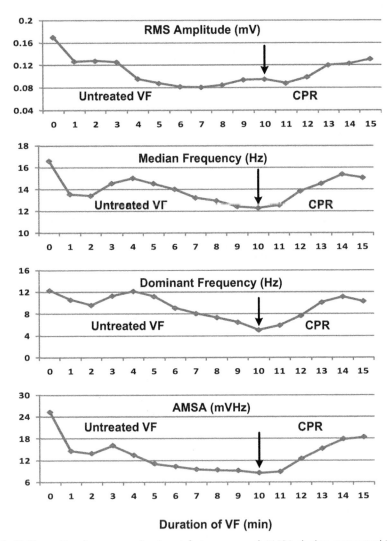

Fig. 2. RMS, median frequency, dominant frequency, and AMSA during untreated VF and CPR in a porcine model of cardiac arrest. CPR was initiated from 10 minutes of VF and lasted for 5 minutes.

obtained. Approaches for optimizing timing of defibrillation include measures based on time domain methods; frequency domain methods, including wavelet-based transformation; nonlinear dynamics methods; and a combination of these methods. **Fig. 2** provides an example of some quantitative measures calculated from the ECG waveforms during untreated VF and CPR.

Time Domain Methods

Earlier investigations using ECG analysis focused on amplitude or voltage of the VF waveform as a predictor of the likelihood of successful defibrillation because this ECG feature reflected myocardial blood flow and energy metabolism.[8,27,28] It has been observed that VF amplitude declines over time, and greater amplitudes, especially after an interval of CPR, are associated with correspondingly greater success of defibrillation.[8,29–33]

Peak-to-peak amplitude, which is defined as the maximum peak-to-peak VF amplitude in a given time window of the ECG signal, is associated with favorable resuscitation outcomes in out-of-hospital CA. Based on the study of Weaver and colleagues,[8] the amplitude of the initial VF waveform was greatest in subjects with witnessed collapse and with shorter intervals from collapse to CPR or from collapse to rescue shock. VF amplitude greater than 0.2 mV is recognized as a predictor of significantly greater likelihood of resuscitation. For subjects with VF amplitude of lower than 0.2 mV, rescue shocks more often result in asystole rather than organized rhythms, and these subjects rarely survive to be admitted to the hospital or discharged alive from the hospital. Survival to discharge increases with amplitude of 0.3 to 0.4 mV and is best for a VF of 0.5 mV or greater.[31,32]

Root-mean-squared (RMS) amplitude is defined as the square root of the mean of the squares of the summed VF amplitude. Initial RMS amplitude of VF is also associated with shock success, ROSC, and discharge from hospital in out-of-hospital CA patients.[34]

Mean and median slope of the ECG waveform, which is defined as the mean and median of the slope of the VF waveform, is also used to predict the defibrillation success and ROSC. Gundersen and colleagues[33] showed that mean probability of ROSC decreases steadily for cases at all initial levels. Regardless of initial level there is a relative decrease in the probability of ROSC of about 23% from 3 to 27 seconds into such a pause by calculating the mean slope using a 2-second window from ECG. Neurauter and coworkers[35] reported a highest area of 0.86 under the receiver operating curve (ROC) by the median slope in the interval 10 to 22 Hz, resulting in a sensitivity of 95% and a specificity of 50% from 197 patients with in-hospital and out-of-hospital CA.

Frequency Domain Methods

Techniques to quantify the component frequencies of the VF signal have employed Fourier and wavelet transformation. Frequency domain features resulting from fast Fourier transform (FFT) analysis of the VF signal include dominant frequency, median frequency, fibrillation power, instantaneous mean frequency, frequency ratio, and amplitude spectrum analysis (AMSA), all of which have been shown to be capable of predicting countershock success.

Dominant frequency, which is defined as the highest power in the VF spectrum, is associated with defibrillation success, ROSC, and survival to hospital discharge in out-of-hospital CA patients.[36–38] Median frequency, which is calculated as the mean of all of the contributing frequencies weighted by the power at each frequency, also serves as a predictor of the success of electrical defibrillation.[29,39] Experimentally, a median frequency of more than 9.14 Hz has 100% sensitivity and 92% specificity in predicting the success of defibrillation.[29,40] Median frequency also correlates with CPPs in animal models as well as human patients and therefore becomes the preferred ECG feature to be used as a predictor of outcome.[27,36,40,41] Other recent investigations have confirmed that there is a relationship between median frequency, dominant frequency, and ROSC after rescue shocks.[42–44]

A refinement of spectrum analysis termed amplitude spectrum analysis (AMSA), calculated as the sum of contributing frequencies weighted by the absolute values of the Fourier transform of the VF signal, has also proved its validity as a predictor for defibrillation outcomes and monitoring the effectiveness of chest compression in animal studies and the clinical scenario.[25,45–47] Retrospective analysis of human ECG records, representing lead 2 equivalent recordings, confirmed the efficacy of this tool in predicting the likelihood that any one electrical shock would have restored a perfusing rhythm during CPR. AMSA values were significantly greater in successful defibrillation, compared to unsuccessful defibrillation. A threshold value of AMSA of 12 mVHz was able to predict the success of each defibrillation attempt with sensitivity and specificity of more than 91% in out-of-hospital CA patients.[48]

Hamprecht and colleagues proposed that fibrillation power is an alternative method of ECG spectral analysis.[49] Defined as the contribution of VF to the power spectral density that eliminated the spectral contribution of artifacts from chest compression, fibrillation power was used to predict the countershock success and matched the established frequency and amplitude analysis both in animal and clinical studies.[36,49]

Sherman[50] proposed a measurement termed frequency ratio, which is defined as the ratio of the power in the high-frequency band from 8 to 24 Hz compared to the power in the low-frequency band from 3 to 5 Hz. Frequency ratio was used to estimate VF duration in an animal study and the results showed that frequency ratio is an improved frequency-based measure of VF duration, with an ROC area of 0.91 at 5 minutes and 0.95 at 7 minutes of VF duration.

Recently, a joint time-frequency approach cited that instantaneous mean frequency (IMF) was used to interpret VF episodes in 204 segments obtained from 13 isolated human hearts. The results suggested that there were significant changes in the spatiotemporal evolution of the frequency. However, IMF has not been evaluated to predict defibrillation outcomes.[51]

Wavelet transform-based time-frequency methods provided a more accurate prediction of rescue shock success in human CA. Energy of the wavelet spectra achieved a sensitivity of 91% and a specificity of 52% for predicting ROSC in the out-of-hospital AED recordings.[52] In another animal experiment, wavelet transform based methodology achieved an overall accuracy of 94% in successfully predicting shock outcomes.[53]

Nonlinear Methods

VF is confirmed to be a complex nonlinear pattern formed by drifting spiral waves of electrical activity that travel across the myocardium and subsequently break down.[54,55] Early debates about whether this chaotic nature can be measured[56,57] have largely settled in favor of some chaotic features for VF.[56,58,59] Analyses of the Hurst exponents and self-similarity dimensions correlate with the duration of VF, which have favored clinical applications.[56] Increased organization in the VF signal is associated with a greater likelihood of shock success. In AED recordings from 75 patients with out-of-hospital CA, the scaling exponent (ScE), which is an estimate of the fractal dimension, was associated with an increased probability of shock success, ROSC, and hospital discharge.[34] Subsequently, several new approaches have been proposed and their effectiveness proved in predicting defibrillation outcomes. One of these animal studies employed $N(\alpha)$ histograms analysis, which was demonstrated to be superior to mean VF frequency analysis.[59]

Angular velocity (AV) is the angle by which an object turns in a certain time. Sherman and colleagues[60] measured the velocity of rotation of the position vector over time by constructing a flat, circular disk-shaped structure in a three-dimensional phase space. Using ScE and AV estimated probability density, VF of less than a 5-minute duration can be identified with 90% sensitivity on the basis of a single 5-second recording of the ECG waveform.

Methods employing entropy measures have also been shown to provide more optimal prediction of ROSC after electrical shock in human VF recordings.[52] Lever and coworkers[61] examined the degree of organization of VF that was induced by electrical stimulation as opposed to occurring clinically due to ischemia or scarring from electrograms recorded by implanted cardiac defibrillators. Using autocorrelation, Shannon entropy, and Kolmogorov entropy, the study confirmed that induced VF had a greater organization than in spontaneous episodes. However, the clinical significance and utility of differences in VF waveform regularity is still unclear.

The logarithm of the absolute correlations (LAC) is a measure based on the roughness of VF waveform. LAC was assessed and compared with the previously published ScE on the ability to predict the duration of VF and the likelihood of ROSC under both experimental and clinical conditions.[62] In a clinical study, the LAC measure was a better predictor of ROSC following initial defibrillation, as reflected by the area under ROC of 0.77 for LAC, compared to 0.57 for ScE.

Detrended fluctuation analysis (DFA), which determines the statistical self-affinity of the VF waveform, is applied to characterize the raw ECG waveform at very short time scales during episodes of cardiac arrhythmias, with the aim to obtain global insight into its dynamic behavior in patients experiencing sudden death.[63] DFA demonstrated a significant difference between patients with successful and unsuccessful defibrillation in a clinical trial that included 155 out-of-hospital CA patients.[64]

Other Methods

Combinations of measurements based on frequency, amplitude, or nonlinear methods may be more predictive of VF outcome than single measurements. For example, a linear combination of amplitude and frequency more accurately predicts ROSC and hospital discharge than either measurement alone.[32] Greater overall accuracy for predicting ROSC in 84 cases of human VF was demonstrated with a combination of total amplitude, peak-to-peak amplitude, proportion of total power in the 2-Hz to 7-Hz range, frequency leakage, and slope of the signal when shocks were applied.[65] In out-of-hospital settings, Eftestøl and colleagues[42,44] analyzed the ability of a linear combination of four spectral features—power, median frequency, spectral flatness, and dominant frequency—recorded by AEDs, from 883 rescue shock attempts on 156 patients.

Neural networks were used by Neurauter and coworkers for single-feature combinations to optimize the prediction of countershock success from 197 patients with in-hospital and out-of-hospital CA.[35] Using frequency band segmentation of human VF ECGs, several single predictive features with high area under ROC (>0.840) were identified. However, combining these single predictive features using neural networks did not further improve outcome prediction in human VF data.

A recent study used genetic programming to fit a relationship between multiple derived measures and defibrillation shock success.[66] It indicated that an optimal algorithm included amplitude, frequency, and nonlinear statistics. This algorithm has not been prospectively tested, however.

LIMITATIONS

Although VF waveform analysis provides satisfactory and encouraging results for optimizing the timing of defibrillation in both animal and clinical studies, considerable concerns still limit implementing currently available methods into clinical devices.

The first limitation involves the use of waveform analysis methods. Concerns preventing the widespread use of VF amplitude as a resuscitation guide include the fact that recording conditions, movement artifact, recording devices, body habitus, and electrode placement may alter measured VF amplitude,[67] even though frequency analysis to assess the VF waveform overcomes some of the problems encountered with amplitude analysis. For example, the technique is robust and less affected by external factors. The power spectra obtained by frequency analysis are similar in simultaneous surface and endocardial ECG leads. Many of the calculations can be performed despite ambient electrical noise or artifact from chest compressions,[43] although the best analyses are still conducted during pauses in chest compressions. There are, however, fundamental problems with FFT analysis. The technique is suitable only for analysis of stationary signals where the waveform does not change. Given the physiologic deterioration in the myocardium during CA, this assumption cannot be extended for VF. The major limitations of the nonlinear methods include the fact that these measurements are numerically intensive to calculate and that they tend to be very sensitive to filtering and noise. As a consequence, these measurements have not been easily incorporated into the present generation of clinical monitors.

The second limitation is that acute ischemic heart disease, such as is present in acute myocardial infarction (AMI) alters VF waveform features.[68] Olasveengen and colleagues[69] demonstrated that AMI patients have a depressed median slope and AMSA compared to patients without AMI during CA. Lever and colleagues[61] confirmed that electrically induced VF had a greater organization than that occurring spontaneously with ischemia. In addition, cardiomyopathy, autonomic dysfunction, and differences in drug therapy make it probable that VF waveform analysis will never demonstrate perfect predictive ability. Because different measurements extract slightly different information from the VF waveform, it is likely that combinations of these measurements will provide superior discriminative ability.[32,65,66] Neurauter and coworkers[35] analyzed 770 ECG recordings of countershock parameters from 197 patients with CA. His study showed that a combination feature employing neural networks does not further improve defibrillation prediction in comparison with the best predictive single features. This result may indicate that an upper limit in outcome prediction using VF waveform analysis in the time and frequency domain has already been reached.

The third limitation is the small number of side-by-side comparisons of various analytical measurements. It is possible that one measurement performs better than another. Only a few papers present results from human data of direct comparisons between various methods.[8,26,34,50] Median frequency appears to be superior to dominant frequency,[29] and AMSA and multiple features of wavelet decomposition appear to be superior to median frequency.[52] Further, methods of filtered ECG features from higher ECG sub-bands, instead of features derived from the main ECG spectrum, have improved the accuracy of shock outcome prediction during CPR.[70] Nonlinear measurements, such as ScE and FDA, are superior to time domain and frequency-based methods.[64] But these comparisons merit further validations with large patient samples.

The final limitation is that all of the existing clinical research has a paucity of prospective validation. Most of the studies have developed measurements by retrospective analysis of electrocardiographic data, and only a few studies have divided the data into training and test sets[32,50] or examined measurements prospectively.[44,51] This lack of validation data and prospective study creates a valid risk of overestimating the performance of each measurement for analyzing human VF. Appropriate validation of each type of measurement will be important before adopting any particular analysis for clinical use.[71]

SUMMARY

There is evidence that features of VF waveforms change over time. Retrospective animal and clinical studies suggest that it is possible to optimize the timing of defibrillation by predicting the success of attempted defibrillation. Higher amplitude, dominant, median and wavelet-based frequency, total fibrillation power and amplitude spectrum area, and lower indices of randomness are all associated with successful defibrillation. Combinations of these measurements may provide a greater predictive power. However, there are still no devices available that are able to analyze the VF waveform in real time and provide reliable information for optimizing the timing of defibrillation. There are no current prospective studies that have identified the optimal measurements for optimizing the timing of defibrillation to improve resuscitation outcome and long-term survival. Therefore, the value of VF waveform analysis to guide defibrillation management is still under investigation.

REFERENCES

1. Cummins RO, Eisenberg MS, Hallstrom AP, et al. Survival of out-of-hospital cardiac arrest with early initiation of cardiopulmonary resuscitaiton. Am J Emerg Med 1985; 3:114–9.
2. Weaver WD, Cobb LA, Hallstrom AP, et al. Considerations for improving survival from out-of-hospital cardiac arrest. Ann Emerg Med 1986;15:1181–6.
3. Eisenberg MS, Copass MK, Hallstrom AP, et al. Treatment of out-of-hospital cardiac arrests with rapid defibrillation by emergency medical technicians. N Engl J Med 1980;302:1379–83.
4. Stults KR, Brown DD, Schug VL, et al. Prehospital defibrillation performed by emergency medical technicians in rural communities. N Engl J Med 1984;310:219–23.
5. European Resuscitation Council. International guidelines 2000 for CPR and ECC—a consensus on science. Resuscitation 2000;46:1–448.
6. Wiggers CJ. The mechanism and nature of ventricular fibrillation. Am Heart J 1940; 20:399–412.
7. Cobb LA, Fahrenbruch CE, Walsh TR, et al. Influence of cardiopulmonary resuscitation prior to defibrillation in patients with out-of-hospital ventricular fibrillation. JAMA 1999;281:1182–8.
8. Weaver WD, Cobb LA, Dennis D, et al. Amplitude of ventricular fibrillation waveform and outcome after cardiac arrest. Ann Intern Med 1985;102:53–5.
9. Ewy GA, Taren D, Bangert J, et al. Comparison of myocardial damage from defibrillation discharges at various dosages. Med Instrum 1980;14:9–12.
10. Warner ED, Dahl C, Ewy GA. Myocardial injury from transthoracic defibrillator countershock. Arch Pathol 1975;99:55–9.
11. Knox MA, Hughes HC Jr, Tyers GF, et al. The induction of myocardial damage by open-chest low-energy countershock. Med Instrum 1980;14:63–6.
12. Valenzuela TD, Roe DJ, Nichol G, et al. Outcomes of rapid defibrillation by security officers after cardiac arrest in casinos. N Engl J Med 2000; 343:1206–9.
13. Wik L, Hansen TB, Fylling F, et al. Delaying defibrillation to give basic cardiopulmonary resuscitation to patients with out-of-hospital ventricular fibrillation. JAMA 2003;289: 1389–95.
14. Berg RA, Hilwig RW, Ewy GA, et al. Precountershock cardiopulmonary resuscitation improves initial response to defibrillation from prolonged ventricular fibrillation: a randomized, controlled swine study. Crit Care Med 2004;32:1352–7.

15. Edelson DP, Abella BS, Kramer-Johansen J, et al. Effects of compression depth and pre-shock pauses predict defibrillation failure during cardiac arrest. Resuscitation 2006;71:137–45.
16. Peatfield RC, Sillett RW, Taylor D, et al. Survival after cardiac arrest in the hospital. Lancet 1977;1:1223–5.
17. DeBard ML. Cardiopulmonary resuscitation: analysis of six years' experience and review of the literature. Ann Emerg Med 1981;10:408–16.
18. Schenenberger RA, von Planta M, von Planta I. Survival after failed out of hospital resuscitation. Are further therapeutic efforts in the emergency department futile? Arch Intern Med 1994;154:2433–7.
19. Xie J, Weil MH, Sun S, et al. High-energy defibrillation increases the severity of postresuscitation myocardial dysfunction. Circulation 1997;96:683–8.
20. Tang W, Weil MH, Sun S, et al. The effects of biphasic waveform design on post resuscitation myocardial function. J Am Coll Cardiol 2004;43:1228–35.
21. Paradis NA, Martin GB, Rivers EP, et al. Coronary perfusion pressure and the return of spontaneous circulation in human cardiopulmonary resuscitation. JAMA 1990;263:1106–13.
22. Gudipati CV, Weil MH, Bisera J, et al. Expired carbon dioxide: a noninvasive monitor of cardiopulmonary resuscitation. Circulation 1988; 77:234–9.
23. Ristagno G, Tang W, Chang YT, et al. The quality of chest compressions during cardiopulmonary resuscitation overrides importance of timing of defibrillation. Chest 2007;132:70–5.
24. Reed MJ, Clegg GR, Robertson CE. Analysing the ventricular fibrillation waveform. Resuscitation 2003;57:11–20.
25. Li Y, Ristagno G, Bisera J, et al. Electrocardiogram waveforms for monitoring effectiveness of chest compression during cardiopulmonary resuscitation. Crit Care Med 2008;36:211–5.
26. Callaway CW, Menegazzi JJ. Waveform analysis of ventricular fibrillation to predict defibrillation. Curr Opin Crit Care 2005;11:192–9.
27. Strohmenger HU, Lindner KH, Brown CG. Analysis of the ventricular fibrillation ECG signal amplitude and frequency parameters as predictors of countershock success in humans. Chest 1997;111:584–9.
28. Noc M, Weil MH, Gazmuri RJ, et al. Ventricular fibrillation voltage as a monitor of the effectiveness of cardiopulmonary resuscitation. J Lab Clin Med 1994;124:421–6.
29. Brown CG, Griffith RF, Van Ligten P, et al. Median frequency: a new parameter for predicting defibrillation success rate. Ann Emerg Med 1991;20:787–9.
30. Dalzell GW, Adgey AA. Determinants of successful transthoracic defibrillation and outcome in ventricular fibrillation. Br Heart J 1991;65:311–6.
31. Callaham M, Braun O, Valentine W, et al. Prehospital cardiac arrest treated by urban first-responders; profile of patient response and prediction of outcome by ventricular fibrillation waveform. Ann Emerg Med 1993;22:1664–77.
32. Monsieurs KG, De Cauwer H, Wuyts FL, et al. A rule for early outcome classification of out-of-hospital cardiac arrest patients presenting with ventricular fibrillation. Resuscitation 1998; 36:37–44.
33. Gundersen K, Kvaløy JT, Kramer-Johansen J, et al. Development of the probability of return of spontaneous circulation in intervals without chest compressions during out-of-hospital cardiac arrest: an observational study. BMC Med 2009;7:6.
34. Callaway CW, Sherman LD, Mosesso VN, et al. Scaling exponent predicts defibrillation success for out-of-hospital ventricular fibrillation cardiac arrest. Circulation 2001; 103:1656–61.

35. Neurauter A, Eftestøl T, Kramer-Johansen J, et al. Prediction of countershock success using single features from multiple ventricular fibrillation frequency bands and feature combinations using neural networks. Resuscitation 2007;73:253–63.
36. Hamprecht FA, Jost D, Ruttimann M, et al. Preliminary results on the prediction of countershock success with fibrillation power. Resuscitation 2001; 50:297–9.
37. Stewart AJ, Allen JD, Adgey AA. Frequency analysis of ventricular fibrillation and resuscitation success. Q J Med 1992;85:761–9.
38. Goto Y, Suzuki I, Inaba H. Frequency of ventricular fibrillation as predictor of one year survival from out-of-hospital cardiac arrests. Am J Cardiol 2003;92:457–9.
39. Brown CG, Dzwonczyk R, Werman HA, et al. Estimating the duration of ventricular fibrillation. Ann Emerg Med 1989;18:1181–5.
40. Strohmenger HU, Lindner KH, Lurie KG, et al. Frequency of ventricular fibrillation as predictor of defibrillation success during cardiac surgery. Anesth Analg 1994;79: 434–8.
41. Brown CG, Dzwonczyk R. Signal analysis of the human electrocardiogram during ventricular fibrillation: frequency and amplitude parameters as predictors of successful countershock. Ann Emerg Med 1996;27:184–8.
42. Eftestøl T, Sunde K, Aase SO, et al. Predicting outcome of defibrillation by spectral characterization and nonparametric classification of ventricular fibrillation in patients with out-of-hospital cardiac arrest. Circulation 2000;102:1523–9.
43. Strohmenger HU, Eftestol T, Sunde K, et al. The predictive value of ventricular fibrillation electrocardiogram signal frequency and amplitude variables in patients with out-of-hospital cardiac arrest. Anesth Analg 2001;93:1428–33.
44. Eftestøl T, Sunde K, Aase SO, et al. Probability of successful defibrillation as a monitor during CPR in out-of-hospital cardiac arrested patients. Resuscitation 2001;48:245–54.
45. Povoas HP, Bisera J. Electrocardiographic waveform analysis for predicting the success of defibrillation. Crit Care Med 2000;28(11 Suppl):N210–1.
46. Marn-Pernat A, Weil MH, Tang W, et al. Optimizing timing of ventricular defibrillation. Crit Care Med 2001;29:2360–5.
47. Povoas HP, Weil MH, Tang W, et al. Predicting the success of defibrillation by electrocardiographic analysis. Resuscitation 2002;53:77–82.
48. Young C, Bisera J, Gehman S, et al. Amplitude spectrum area: measuring the probability of successful defibrillation as applied to human data. Crit Care Med 2004;32(9 Suppl):S356–8.
49. Hamprecht FA, Achleitner U, Krismer AC, et al. Fibrillation power, an alternative method of ECG spectral analysis for prediction of countershock success in a porcine model of ventricular fibrillation. Resuscitation 2001;50:287–96.
50. Sherman LD. The frequency ratio: an improved method to estimate ventricular fibrillation duration based on Fourier analysis of the waveform. Resuscitation 2006; 69:479–86.
51. Umapathy K, Massé S, Sevaptsidis E, et al. Spatiotemporal frequency analysis of ventricular fibrillation in explanted human hearts. IEEE Trans Biomed Eng 2009;56: 328–35.
52. Watson JN, Uchaipichat N, Addison PS, et al. Improved prediction of defibrillation success for out-of-hospital VF cardiac arrest using wavelet transform methods. Resuscitation 2004;63:269–75.
53. Umapathy K, Krishnan S, Masse S, et al. Optimizing cardiac resuscitation outcomes using wavelet analysis. Conf Proc IEEE Eng Med Biol Soc 2009;6761–4.
54. Jalife J, Gray R. Drifting vortices of electrical waves underlie ventricular fibrillation in the rabbit heart. Acta Physiol Scand 1996;157:123–31.

55. Panfilov AV. Spiral break up as a model of ventricular fibrillation. Chaos 1998;8:57–64.
56. Sherman L, Callaway CW, Menegazzi JJ. Ventricular fibrillation exhibits dynamical properties and self-similarity. Resuscitation 2000;47:163–73.
57. Eftestøl T, Wik L, Sunde K, et al. Effects of cardiopulmonary resuscitation on predictors of ventricular fibrillation defibrillation success during out-of hospital cardiac arrest. Circulation 2004;110:10–5.
58. Small M, Yu D, Harrison RG, et al. Deterministic nonlinearity in ventricular fibrillation. Chaos 2000;10:268–77.
59. Amann A, Achleitner U, Antretter H, et al. Analysing ventricular fibrillation ECG-signals and predicting defibrillation success during cardiopulmonary resuscitation employing N(alpha)-histograms. Resuscitation 2001;50:77–85.
60. Sherman LD, Flagg A, Callaway CW, et al. Angular velocity: a new method to improve prediction of ventricular fibrillation duration. Resuscitation 2004;60:79–90.
61. Lever NA, Newall EG, Larsen PD. Differences in the characteristics of induced and spontaneous episodes of ventricular fibrillation. Europace 2007;9:1054–8.
62. Sherman LD, Rea TD, Waters JD, et al. Logarithm of the absolute correlations of the ECG waveform estimates duration of ventricular fibrillation and predicts successful defibrillation. Resuscitation 2008;78:346–54.
63. Rodriguez E, Lerma C, Echeverria JC, et al. ECG scaling properties of cardiac arrhythmias using detrended fluctuation analysis. Physiol Meas 2008;29:1255–66.
64. Lin LY, Lo MT, Ko PC, et al. Detrended fluctuation analysis predicts successful defibrillation for out-of-hospital ventricular fibrillation cardiac arrest. Resuscitation 2010;81:297–301.
65. Callaway CW, Sherman LD, Menegazzi JJ, et al. Scaling structure of electrocardiographic waveform during prolonged ventricular fibrillation in swine. Pacing Clin Electrophysiol 2000; 23:180–91.
66. Podbregar M, Kovaib M, Podbregar-Marc A, et al. Predicting defibrillation success by 'genetic' programming in patients with out-of-hospital cardiac arrest. Resuscitation 2003;57:153–9.
67. Indik JH, Peters CM, Donnerstein RL, et al. Direction of signal recording affects waveform characteristics of ventricular fibrillation in humans undergoing defibrillation testing during ICD implantation. Resuscitation 2008;78:38–45.
68. Indik JH, Shanmugasundaram M, Allen D, et al. Predictors of resuscitation outcome in a swine model of VF cardiac arrest: a comparison of VF duration, presence of acute myocardial infarction and VF waveform. Resuscitation 2009;80:1420–3.
69. Olasveengen TM, Eftestol T, Gundersen K, et al. Acute ischemic heart disease alters ventricular fibrillation waveform characteristics in out-of hospital cardiac arrest. Resuscitation 2009;80:412–7.
70. Neurauter A, Eftestøl T, Kramer-Johansen J, et al. Improving countershock success prediction during cardiopulmonary resuscitation using ventricular fibrillation features from higher ECG frequency bands. Resuscitation 2008;79:453–9.
71. American Heart Association. 2010 American Heart Association Guidelines for Cardiopulmonary Resuscitation and Emergency Cardiovascular Care. Part 6: electrical therapies: automated external defibrillators, defibrillation, cardioversion, and pacing. Circulation 2010;122;S706–19.

Emergency Cardiopulmonary Bypass: A Promising Rescue Strategy for Refractory Cardiac Arrest

David F. Gaieski, MD[a,b],*, Manuel Boller, Dr med. vet, MTR[b,c],
Lance B. Becker, MD[a,b]

KEYWORDS
- Sudden cardiac arrest • Cardiopulmonary resuscitation
- Cardiopulmonary bypass • Extracorporeal membrane oxygenation

Emergency cardiopulmonary bypass (ECPB) has been investigated experimentally and clinically as an advanced resuscitation method that may rescue patients with refractory cardiac arrest or cardiogenic shock unresponsive to traditional medical interventions. By diverting blood flow from the patient to an extracorporeal heart and lung system capable of providing full cardiac output, ECPB can provide blood flow and gas exchange to the patient when there is not the capability of the patient's heart or lungs to sustain these functions intrinsically. This method extends the time window for successful interventions to correct the underlying pathophysiology leading to arrest or shock.

Background of Cardiac Arrest and Post Cardiac Arrest Syndrome

There is no universal reporting system for cardiopulmonary arrests in the United States. However, it has been estimated that approximately 350,000 arrests occur each year, with 50% happening out-of-hospital and the other half to patients in a hospital setting.[1] Less than 40% of these patients have return of spontaneous circulation (ROSC), and mortality for those with ROSC exceeds 60%.[2] The 2010 American Heart Association (AHA) guidelines for cardiopulmonary resuscitation (CPR)

The authors have nothing to disclose.

[a] Department of Emergency Medicine, Perelman School of Medicine, University of Pennsylvania, 3400 Spruce Street, Ground Ravdin, Philadelphia, PA 19104, USA
[b] Center for Resuscitation Science, University of Pennsylvania, 125 South 31st Street, TRL Suite 1200, Philadelphia, PA 19104, USA
[c] Section of Critical Care, Department of Clinical Studies, School of Veterinary Medicine, University of Pennsylvania, 3900 Delancey Street, Philadelphia, PA 19104, USA
* Corresponding author. Department of Emergency Medicine, Perelman School of Medicine, University of Pennsylvania, 3400 Spruce Street, Ground Ravdin, Philadelphia, PA 19104.
E-mail address: David.Gaieski@uphs.upenn.edu

0749-0704/12/$ – see front matter © 2012 Elsevier Inc. All rights reserved.

emphasize high-quality CPR including early defibrillation, chest compressions at the correct rate and depth, and appropriately sequenced advanced airway management, intravenous (IV) access, and drug administration to maximize the percentage of arrest patients achieving sustained ROSC.

Patients with ROSC after cardiac arrest fall on a continuum of neurologic injury sustained during the arrest ranging from those who are awake, alert, and neurologically intact to those who are comatose, unresponsive, and potentially neurologically devastated. Patients who manifest organ dysfunction after cardiac arrest have post-cardiac arrest syndrome (PCAS) and need targeted therapy to optimize outcomes. These therapies center around therapeutic hypothermia (TH), which has been demonstrated to improve survival and neurologic outcomes in PCAS patients.

The Three-Phase Model of Cardiac Arrest

One of the main factors that dictates the severity of the PCAS is the length of time from collapse to ROSC. In 2002, Weisfeldt and Becker[3] proposed a three-phase time-sensitive model of cardiac arrests caused by shockable rhythms, suggesting that patients pass through sequential periods of arrest where different interventions should take priority. The first phase is the electrical phase, lasting approximately 4 minutes, during which defibrillation takes precedence. Approximately 5 minutes after the start of arrest the patient enters the circulatory phase, in which high-quality chest compressions take precedence over defibrillation. The notion of restoring some perfusion first followed by defibrillation is an attempt to restore some myocardial oxygen delivery, adenosine triphosphate (ATP), and action potentials so that electrical defibrillation attempts can be more successful. After the circulatory phase comes the metabolic phase wherein chest compression and defibrillation alone simply will not save the vast majority of patients. The endogenous injury from ischemia and no or low flow during the arrest accrues to a degree that it comes to dominate intraarrest physiology. At this point it is much more difficult to achieve ROSC, and most patients are pronounced dead. Survival and neurologic function decrease with increasing length of CPR and decreasing quality of advanced cardiac life support (ACLS) techniques. ROSC is difficult to achieve with increased length of resuscitation because a vicious cycle ensues: → low cardiac output → further ischemia → refractory ventricular fibrillation (VF) or recurrent arrest → worsened metabolic phase.[4,5]

Role of Emergency Cardiopulmonary Bypass

ECPB seems to have the best potential for patients in the lethal metabolic phase of cardiac arrest during which chest compressions and defibrillation fail the vast majority of the time. ECPB seems to be effective in three broad categories of clinical arrest: (1) patients for whom cardiac arrest would not be expected to be reversed by traditional ACLS, such as profound hypothermia or overwhelming drug intoxication; (2) patients with cardiac arrest refractory to standard ACLS, such as those in the metabolic phase or who have failed to respond to ACLS; or (3) for salvage of patients who achieve ROSC but show signs of postarrest deterioration such as profound cardiogenic shock or, less commonly, refractory hypoxemia from postarrest pulmonary injury. The fundamental principles behind ECPB are to provide exogenous full-body circulation and gas exchange to patients who can no longer adequately perform these functions endogenously. This method allows an extended window of investigation and intervention to determine the cause of the arrest and take the necessary steps to restore adequate endogenous organ function.

DEFINITION OF TERMS/CONCEPTS/TYPES OF EXTRACORPOREAL CIRCULATION

A number of different options for extracorporeal circulation exist including extracorporeal membrane oxygenation (ECMO), ECPB, continuous venovenous hemofiltration (CVVH), hemodialysis, and plasmapheresis. These modalities vary depending on their primary function: circulation, gas exchange, or filtration of electrolytes and other metabolically active substances. For this review the authors focus almost exclusively on ECPB, which can provide adequate circulation and gas exchange to replace native heart and lung function.

Percutaneous Cardiopulmonary Support Systems

Percutaneous cardiopulmonary support (PCPS) is a general term for portable battery-powered heart-lung machines, which can provide extracorporeal circulation in a number of venues for a variety of reasons.

Emergency cardiopulmonary bypass

ECPB uses a venous cannula to aspirate blood, usually via a femoral site, from the venous circulation to a centrifugal or, less commonly, a roller pump acting as an extracorporeal heart and to a membrane oxygenator, acting as an extracorporeal lung, before returning the blood to the body through an arterial cannula to be distributed throughout the body.

Extracorporeal membrane oxygenation

ECMO is a method of providing artificial cardiac or pulmonary support or both and is frequently used as a rescue strategy in the pediatric population. Like ECPB, it is initiated by placement of percutaneous cannulae, often via the femoral vasculature. ECMO has two main types: VA, or venoarterial, and VV, or venovenous. Whereas VA-ECMO provides both cardiac and pulmonary support, VV-ECMO provides only pulmonary support and is primarily used for treatment of patients with severe lung injury such as acute respiratory distress syndrome.

Continuous venovenous hemofiltration

CVVH is a technique of removing blood from a patient's venous circulation, using a pump to pass the blood over a convection filter utilizing a pressure gradient, and removing specific solutes from the blood before returning the filtered blood to the patient's venous circulation. It has been used in cardiac arrest patients to remove endotoxin and other inflammatory mediators from the PCAS patient's blood.[6] However, CVVH cannot be used to provide cardiac or pulmonary support.

Hemodialysis

Hemodialysis provides similar clinical interventions as CVVH but uses dialysate to produce diffusion of solutes across a semipermeable membrane. Like CVVH, hemodialysis is typically used to remove creatinine and urea along with other waste products of metabolism from the blood of patients with either acute or chronic renal failure. It provides no cardiac or pulmonary support and cannot be used as a primary therapy for treatment of refractory cardiac arrest. However, hemodialysis can be used as an adjunct therapy in patients postarrest.

Plasmapheresis

Plasmapheresis is typically performed by removing blood via a venous cannula, centrifuging the blood to separate the plasma from the cells in the blood, and then removing antibodies and other disease-causing proteins before returning the filtered plasma to the patient. Many autoimmune disorders including Guillain-Barré syndrome, thrombotic thrombocytopenic purpura, and myasthenia gravis are treated by plasmapheresis. However, plasmapheresis is not typically used to treat cardiac arrest patients.

Therapeutic hypothermia

TH is the only therapy that has been systematically demonstrated to improve outcomes in comatose survivors of cardiac arrest and has become the standard of care in the treatment of neurologically injured PCAS patients. A number of different approaches to the induction of TH are available including induction with IV-chilled saline infusion, surface cooling with ice bags, rapid immersion systems, surface-cooling wraps, IV cooling catheters, and maintenance of TH with surface or IV devices. Importantly, TH can be induced and maintained using ECPB, ECMO, or CVVH circuits, and these have been used to deliver TH to postarrest patients. If ECPB is used as a rescue strategy for refractory arrest patients, most centers now advocate using ECPB together with TH.

Ischemia/reperfusion and reperfusion injury

During ischemia there is no blood flow or oxygen delivered to the tissues. CPR attempts to convert this no-flow state into a low-flow state until native circulation is restored. Whereas ROSC is the immediate goal of resuscitation, there is much evidence that some of the tissue injury observed is due to factors within the reperfusion phase. In other words, although the ischemia causes injury, the injury may be reversible depending on the conditions of reperfusion.

BRIEF HISTORY OF EMERGENCY CARDIOPULMONARY BYPASS

ECPB grew out of the initial use of cardiopulmonary bypass for surgical repair of cardiac defects. After conceptual and developmental advances in the early part of the 20th century, the first clinical applications of extracorporeal circulation were undertaken in the 1950s.[7] As early as 1937, Gibbon[8] proposed the idea of using cardiopulmonary bypass (CPB) to treat massive pulmonary embolism. The first known CPB-assisted operation was performed by Dr Clarence Dennis at the University of Wisconsin in 1951. Refinements in pump function leading to less blood damage and improvements in membrane function producing better gas exchange have allowed CPB to be used on a daily basis at hundreds of institutions around the world.

Brief Introduction to Reperfusion Injury

Understanding of reperfusion injury after ischemia continues to grow but remains incomplete. A fundamental question involved in ischemia and reperfusion is, "When does cell death occur?" Is cell death irreversible after a period of ischemia, or at the time of onset of reperfusion (ROSC) are cells still salvageable and cell death occurs during reperfusion? Events of prolonged ischemia set the biochemical stage for reperfusion injury: low ATP levels, elevated reactive oxygen/nitrogen species, reduced electron transport cytochromes, and intracellular calcium (Ca^{2+}) overload. Into this dangerously primed biochemical medium current reperfusion practice introduces sudden reoxygenation, creating a burst of new reactive oxygen species, lipid oxidation, mitochondrial Ca^{2+} overload, mitochondrial permeability transition, and the systemic amplification of destructive biochemical cascades. Metabolic strategies to attenuate reperfusion injury could in theory prevent some of these destructive cascades while allowing restoration of blood flow and promoting long-term neurologically intact survival. Groundwork for this concept comes from the laboratories of

Buckberg and colleagues.[9,10] They proposed controlled reperfusion using a high osmolarity, low Ca^{2+} cocktail of antioxidants, which includes neuroprotective agents and leukocyte filtration to prevent reperfusion injury in a number of animal models and diverse types of ischemic injuries. This concept of reperfusion injury is vital to understanding the use of ECPB, because ECPB has the potential to control the conditions of reperfusion and reduce reperfusion injury. Thus, ECPB plus a strategy to control reperfusion injury is of growing scientific interest.

RATIONALE FOR ECPB IN CPR

The rationale for studying ECPB in CPR settings includes the following:

- A growing literature to support its effectiveness.
- In expert hands, can be rapidly initiated to maintain circulation.
- Bridge until effective native cardiac output is restored.

Emergency Department Patients May Be Ideal ECPB Candidates

In some cases, emergency department (ED) patients are perfect candidates for the novel ECPB resuscitation strategy: They are typically healthy at the time of their arrest and actively engaged in life, the cause of arrest is more likely to be cardiac, the initial rhythm is more often a shockable rhythm than in patients who arrest in a hospital setting, many out-of-hospital cardiac arrests receive bystander CPR, and automated external defibrillators are often used, providing early defibrillation. All of these actions increase the likelihood of the patient having ROSC and being a candidate for postarrest care; similarly, these actions prolong the period of arrest prior to irreversible neurologic injury and can allow patients still in arrest to be salvageable by alternative resuscitation strategies on ED arrival. However, a significant percentage of these patients do not achieve ROSC by conventional means and are, in the overwhelming majority of cases, pronounced dead at the location of the arrest or in the ED. In one sense these patients are "too healthy to die," and alternative resuscitation strategies are desperately required.

Therapeutic Hypothermia with ECPB

Another attractive aspect of ECPB as a rescue strategy for patients with refractory cardiac arrest is that ECPB is an efficient and rapid means of delivering TH. Blood removed from a patient's venous system can be rapidly cooled to a chosen temperature prior to reintroduction into the arterial side of the patient's circulation. Using this approach, a patient can be cooled from the presenting temperature (often ~ 36°C) to the target temperature for therapeutic cooling (most commonly 33°C) over 20 to 30 minutes.[11]

EXPERIMENTAL EVIDENCE SUPPORTING IMPLEMENTATION OF EMERGENCY CARDIOPULMONARY BYPASS

Animal models in species such as rats, dogs, and swine have been fundamental to the development of CPB and ECMO.[12] In contrast to a vast literature on CPB, only a small number of studies have been published on the use of extracorporeal circulation technology as a resuscitative measure after cardiac arrest.

ECPB as an Alternative Method to Improve Survival from Prolonged Cardiac Arrest

More than two decades ago the Pittsburgh group led by Safar[13] conducted a series of dog studies to systematically address two important questions: (a) Would ECPB resuscitation be better than traditional advanced life support (ALS)? and (b) What is the longest duration of arrest that could be survived? Reich and colleagues[14] examined the cardiac resuscitatability with ECPB in dogs after escalating durations of untreated VF. After 15 and 20 minutes of no-flow cardiac arrest, all dogs were successfully defibrillated, weaned off normothermic ECPB within 4 hours, and maintained stable spontaneous circulation to the end of the study. After 30 minutes from arrest all animals achieved ROSC, but only 5 of 10 dogs could be weaned off ECPB, and 100% deteriorated hemodynamically prior to the end of the study period. After 15 minutes from cardiac arrest all animals achieved normal neurologic function after 4 days, whereas this was not the case for any animals after longer arrest durations.[13] In addition, the investigators demonstrated that basic life support (BLS; chest compressions) could markedly prolong the window of opportunity for success-ful ECPB.[15] In these experiments, 2 minutes of untreated VF was followed by 30 minutes of BLS before ECPB was instituted. All animals achieved ROSC, and 70% survived neurologically intact to 72 hours. When ECPB was replaced with ALS, only 20% of the animals survived neurologically intact to 72 hours, thus demonstrating superiority of ECPB over standard ALS, perhaps due to better coronary perfusion pressure.[16]

The Pittsburgh group also conducted a series of fundamental experiments directly comparing conventional CPR and ECPB after various lengths of untreated (no-flow) VF, the results of which were summarized concisely by Safar and colleagues[13] in 1990 and are briefly outlined here. These studies collectively suggest ECPB to be superior to ALS. For example, after 20 minutes of no-flow VF, ALS restored stable ROSC in 7 of 9 dogs, whereas ECPB did so in 13 of 13 animals and produced a more favorable hemodynamic profile.

In a study to better simulate the out-of-hospital cardiac arrest (OHCA) scenario, 4 minutes of no-flow VF was followed by 30 minutes of BLS, and after these 34 minutes of cardiac arrest either ALS or ECPB was instituted. All animals in the ECPB group achieved ROSC versus 5 of 10 animals in the CPR-ALS group. In addition 70% of ECPB-resuscitated animals achieved intact neurologic function after 4 days, indicat-ing that good neurologic outcome can be achieved with ECPB support after more than 30 minutes of high-quality CPR-BLS.

Refinement of ECPB

Physical optimization

ECPB-based strategies allow control of both physical and pharmacologic conditions under which reperfusion takes place. For example, TH improves survival when used with ECPB. Ao and colleagues[17] compared the impact of hypothermic (33°C) versus normothermic (37°C) ECPB of 24 hours duration followed by 72 hours of intensive care on cardiovascular and neurologic recovery after 15 minutes of untreated VF. There was a pronounced treatment benefit of TH with regard to survival (6 of 7 vs normothermia, 0 of 8), neurologic function, hippocampal CA1 neuron degeneration, and myocardial infarction area. In a second study, the same investigators demon-strated that very rapid cooling (1.6 ± 0.8 minutes) compared with slow cooling (49.5 ± 12.1 minutes) to target temperature of 33°C may not have an impact on survival but improved functional and histologic neurologic outcome.[13,18] The Pittsburgh group systematically evaluated the value of ECPB and hypothermia for resuscitation from prolonged cardiac arrest; ECPB was found to allow for rapid cooling to 33°C within 30 seconds of reperfusion and was associated with improved neurologic outcomes compared with normothermic reperfusion.[13,19]

The authors found in their own rat ECPB model (**Fig. 1**) that bypass-administered cooling affords significant neurologic and survival benefit after asphyxial cardiac

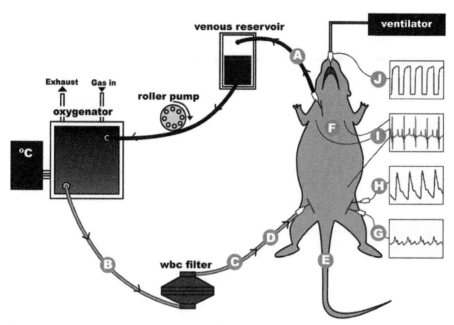

Fig. 1. The experimental setup of a simplified rodent ECPB model. The right atrium is cannulated with a 14-G cannula via the external jugular vein for venous outflow, whereas the arterial return occurs via the right femoral artery. A miniaturized membrane oxygenator is used for blood oxygenation and carbon dioxide removal. Total circuit volume is 30 mL. The letters indicate the location of monitoring components: (A) central venous oxygen saturation, (B) circuit pressure sensor, (C) oxygen partial pressure sensor, (D) circuit temperature, (E) rectal temperature, (F) esophageal temperature, (G) central venous pressure, (H) arterial blood pressure, (I) electrocardiography, (J) capnography.

arrest when compared with a normothermic strategy.[20] In this study, Sprague-Dawley rats were resuscitated with ECPB after 8 minutes of normothermic cardiac arrest. With the initiation of bypass, animals were either cooled to 30°C or 34°C, or they were maintained at 37°C. Survival after ECPB resuscitation in different groups demonstrated the dramatic impact of hypothermia on 72-hour survival, with no animals surviving after normothermic ECPB, and 8 of 10 and 6 of 10 animals survived when treated with moderate and mild hypothermia, respectively (**Fig. 2**). However, it seems that cooling can be even more protective when it is initiated during the intraarrest period prior to reperfusion.[13] Such intraarrest hypothermia preceding initiation of ECPB was studied by Nozari and colleagues,[21] who compared early versus delayed cooling in a canine OHCA model. Rapid cooling to 34°C was either initiated very early prior to ROSC or was delayed by 10 minutes. Delaying cooling by only 10 minutes reduced survival from 78% to 13%. Moreover, the majority of the survivors (5 of 7) in the early cooling group had good neurologic outcomes at 72 hours. These earlier findings were corroborated by subsequent studies in the same laboratory that demonstrated the remarkable neuroprotective effects of early intraarrest (prereperfusion) cooling by aortic flush followed by ECPB resuscitation in a canine hemorrhagic arrest model.[22–24] Further work on the protective effect of intraarrest cooling demonstrated that rapid induction of profound hypothermia (10°C tympanic temperature) after exsanguination cardiac arrest and subsequent resuscitation with ECPB

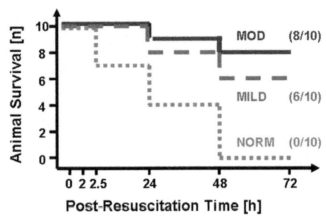

Fig. 2. Survival 72 hours after ECPB resuscitation from 8 minutes of asphyxial cardiac arrest in a rat model. The Kaplan-Meier plot demonstrates the markedly superior survival rate in rats treated with mild (*MILD*) or moderate (*MOD*) hypothermic reperfusion and postresuscitation hypothermia for 8 hours, compared with those maintained normothermic (*NORM*) throughout the study period of 3 days. (*From* Han F, Boller M, Guo W, et al. A rodent model of emergency cardiopulmonary bypass resuscitation with different temperatures after asphyxial cardiac arrest. Resuscitation 2010;81;93–9; with permission.)

allowed no-flow times with intact neurologic survival of up to 120 minutes in dogs.[25] This principle of prolonged cold preserved no-flow cardiac arrest with delayed controlled ECPB resuscitation, known as suspended animation or emergency preservation and resuscitation, illustrates the powerful protective resuscitative potential of TH combined with ECPB.[26] In addition to hypothermia, other physical modifications of ECPB-based reperfusion were shown to exert benefit. Hypertensive hemodilution achieved by administration of norepinephrine and dextran to a mean arterial pressure (MAP) greater than 140 mm Hg and a hematocrit of 20% and paired with ECPB was shown to prevent the occurrence of postarrest cerebral hypoperfusion and may improve neurologic function.[27]

Neuroprotection during experimental CPB has also been reported in pulsatile bypass studies when compared with nonpulsatile bypass,[28,29] with an improvement in cerebral blood flow,[30,31] better autoregulation,[32] and reduced markers for cerebral hypoxia.[33–35] Moreover, Anstadt and colleagues[36] tested the influence of pulsatile versus nonpulsatile ECPB on neurologic outcome measures in a dog model of prolonged (12.5 minutes) VF arrest[36] and reported that nonpulsatile flow produced more severe hippocampal CA1 neuron dropout, more frequent ischemic changes in the caudate nucleus and cerebral cortex, and a trend toward more severe neurologic functional deficit 7 days after resuscitation. Although promising, clearly more study is required on the use of pulsatile-flow versus continuous-flow ECPB.

Pharmacologic optimization

ECPB also provides an opportunity to exert considerable control over chemical or pharmacologic constituents of the reperfusate with the target of mitigating ischemia and reperfusion injury. Several experimental studies demonstrate the ability of some drugs to improve outcome even when these drugs are given with the reperfusion after ischemia (ie, thereby preventing reperfusion injury). However, there is conflicting literature in this important area. For example, in early reperfusion the sodium hydrogen exchange antiporter opens after ischemia and leads to sodium influx and contributes to intracellular Ca^{2+} overload. There are studies that show both the effectiveness and noneffectiveness of sodium hydrogen exchange inhibitors with initiation of ECPB for resuscitation from prolonged cardiac arrest nonresponsive to ACLS.[37] Similarly, the effect of an N-methyl-D-aspartate antagonist was examined in a canine cardiac arrest and ECPB model in order to minimize excitotoxicity associated with cerebral ischemia and reperfusion, but no protective effect was evident.[22] These studies suggest that these agents when used alone in reperfusion have limited effectiveness against the cumulative injury.

Whereas most single agents fail to protect when used during reperfusion after ischemia, there is more enthusiasm for the use of combination therapy with multiple compounds added to the bypass circuit prime to improve outcome. The scientific rationale for these cocktail components is that because multiple destructive pathways are active during reperfusion, multiple agents are required to correct the complex intertwined injury cascades that unfold during and after ischemia and reperfusion. Therefore, such treatments lead to an overall enhanced additive or synergistic benefit effect compared with what would be achievable with single-agent therapy alone. Combinations of agents in the literature include the use of Ca^{2+} chelators or Ca^{2+} channel blockers added to the bypass prime to counteract intracellular Ca^{2+} overload during reperfusion.[38] Magnesium sulfate was examined as an additional method to antagonize the intracellular effects of Ca^{2+} as well as for its neuroprotective potential after ischemia and reperfusion.[38,39] The nonbicarbonate buffer tromethamine (THAM) was added in a dose that limits acidemia during reperfusion yet does not lead to normalization of the pH, because both severe acidosis and overzealous buffer administration were implicated in increased neuronal and myocardial injury after ischemia and reperfusion.[38,40–42] Hetastarch or dextran was added empirically to the CPB prime in many experimental ECPB studies to limit a reduction in colloid osmotic pressure and to combat interstitial edema formation.[13] Reperfusion from global ischemia after cardiac arrest as well as the use of ECPB itself leads to endothelial activation and vascular leakage.[43] Mannitol to reduce intracellular edema in addition to its postulated radical scavenging effects was also a frequent component of controlled reperfusion cocktails.[38] Complement and leukocyte activation and systemic inflammation are relevant pathophysiologic mechanisms after resuscitation from cardiac arrest but do also occur with CPB and cardiac surgery.[44–46] Thus, filter-leukodepletion to remove the vast majority of leukocytes from whole blood containing prime and integration of leukodepletion filters into the ECPB circuit have been included in protective reperfusion strategies.[47–49] In large animal models, post-cardiac arrest reperfusion combined with leukocyte depletion led to reduction of oxidative injury and complement C5b-9 (membrane attack complex) and was shown to improve functional myocardial and neurologic recovery.[47–49] Finally, packed red blood cells have been used in the bypass prime to increase oxygen transport capacity of the reperfusate.[37]

An example of the effectiveness of this cocktail approach can be seen in a piglet model of deep (19°C) prolonged (90 minutes) hypothermic cardiac arrest. Allen and colleagues[47,48] compared a controlled, combinatorial global reperfusion and rewarming strategy (normoxia, citrate, magnesium sulfate, pH-stat, mannitol, leukodepletion blood prime, Na+/H+ exchange inhibitor) with what was considered usual clinical practice (unmodified blood prime, 100% oxygen, alpha-stat). The animals receiving the cocktail had lower release of conjugated dienes (lipid peroxidation), endothelin-1 (vascular injury), and creatinine kinase (cellular injury) and better neurologic deficit scores. Trummer and colleagues[38] described the use of a controlled reperfusion strategy in a swine model of prolonged sudden cardiac arrest. In this study the bypass prime (cocktail) included lidocaine, citrate, magnesium sulfate, mannitol, and pH-stat. Next to the bypass prime, the study controlled physical aspects of reperfusion, which included initial low-flow and low blood pressure (30–40 mm Hg) reperfusion followed by full-flow CPB, fast induction of moderate hypothermia (30°C), and pH-stat to increase cerebral blood flow. Also, leukodepletion filters were included into the arterial bypass line. Conditions were controlled for 60 minutes. All animals (7 of 7) were successfully resuscitated with the cocktail versus zero animals getting standard CPR and ACLS. In addition, good neurologic functional recovery was observed in 6 of 7 animals.

There are many unknowns in the optimal reperfusion conditions following prolonged ischemia, including the proper level of reoxygenation to target after resuscitation. Proper oxygen level during reperfusion and avoidance of hyperoxia has been associated with reduced postresuscitation oxidative injury in experimental and clinical studies.[50–52] It is possible that avoidance of early hyperoxic reperfusion during ECPB may improve myocardial and neurologic function. Yoshitake and colleagues[53] demonstrated that in a canine model of prolonged VF (15 minutes), hypoxemic ECPB worsens outcome despite maintained blood flow. However, experimental studies are awaited to define a target partial pressure of oxygen in arterial blood (Pao_2) level during ECPB that is both safe and effective.[53] Execution of such studies may be hampered by the lack of correlation between arterial and tissue normoxia or hyperoxia after ischemia and reperfusion injury and by technological limitations in determining actual levels of tissue oxygenation. The ideal oxygenation level following ischemia remains unknown.

Limitation of Animal Models

As much as cardiac arrest and ECPB studies are designed to mimic reality, subjects are anesthetized healthy adolescent and single-gender animals.[54,55] This homogeneity leads to problems with the external validity and generalizability of the models,[56] because attributes of the OHCA human population include older age, 1:2 female-to-male ratio, numerous comorbidities (eg, coronary artery disease, hypertension, diabetes mellitus), and highly variable cardiac arrest to CPR (no-flow) and CPR to ROSC (low-flow) intervals.[57] Inhalant anesthetics that are a frequent part of experimental animal studies but are rarely part of human periarrest management are capable of inducing marked dose-dependent preconditioning and can lead to protection even hours after discontinuation of anesthesia when the vast majority of the anesthetic is washed out.[58]

In ECPB models, prearrest heparinization is universally used to prevent clot formation in catheters placed during instrumentation of the animals, whereas this is rarely the case in humans. Findings in a canine ECPB model suggested that not only the presence or absence of heparin pretreatment but also the heparin dose may impact the resuscitation success.[59] In that study, animals pretreated with 700 U/kg unfractionated heparin had better short-term hemodynamic outcome and survival rate (6 of 6 vs 2 of 6) compared with those animals treated with 200 U/kg. Moreover, the small size of some animals such as rats may be a benefit in many aspects, such as considerable cost savings and ease of handling compared with swine or dog models, but postresuscitation care is limited and dissimilar to contemporary medical critical care. This difference may limit the survivability of more severe injuries because of factors that would not necessarily be outcome-limiting in humans.

INITIAL CLINICAL TRIALS

ECPB is a new concept, with the bulk of human literature reported only during the last 12 years. There are some earlier studies investigating ECPB that are available only in Japanese-language literature. Preliminary English-language studies on treating a heterogeneous patient populations including cardiac arrest, refractory shock, and complicated myocardial infarction began to appear as early as 1976; however, the majority of reports on the human use of ECPB begin in 1999.[60-62] The first major English-language publication of an investigation of ECPB as an alternate resuscitation strategy for patients in refractory cardiac arrest was published in *Chest* in 1999.[63] In this pilot study, 10 VF patients between the ages of 14 and 65 were treated with ECPB. Inclusion criteria were patients with witnessed cardiac arrest (OHCA or in ED) of less than 30 minutes duration unresponsive to ACLS who had been intubated, defibrillated up to three times, and received at least one dose of epinephrine (1 mg) but remained in VF. CPB was initiated by an on-call ED research team consisting of emergency physicians with laboratory experience in deployment of CPB by a femoral-femoral route who were assisted by certified perfusion technologists. They used a Bard PCPS device. A 77-cm, 20 French venous catheter was placed with its tip in the right atrium and a 36-cm, 20 French arterial catheter was placed with its tip in the iliac artery. Blood was removed from the venous system and passed through a pump, membrane oxygenator, and heat exchanger before returning to the patient via the arterial cannula.

For the 10 cases described in this study, the mean time to pump was 32.0 ± 13.6 minutes, and the mean time on ECPB was 229 ± 111 minutes. All of the patients (10 of 10) had ROSC, 70% were weaned from CPB, and 60% survived discharge from ED to intensive care unit (ICU) admission. The mean cardiac output prior to weaning from ECPB was 4.09 ± 1.03 L/min. However, none (0 of 10) regained an acceptable level of neurologic function and none (0 of 10) survived to hospital discharge. The average time from ED arrival to death was 48 hours.

The investigators concluded, "The results of this study support the idea that CPB alone is not enough to ensure neurologically intact survival after resuscitation from prolonged cardiac arrest unresponsive to ACLS." In addition, they noted the need for more systematic treatment of PCAS: "With increased awareness of the post-resuscitation disease and therapy aimed at alleviating ischemia reperfusion injury, more success with CPB as a resuscitative tool may be expected."

The same year, Younger and colleagues[64] published the results of their case series of refractory arrest patients treated with ECPB, which they termed *extracorporeal cardiopulmonary resuscitation* (ECPR). ECPR was attempted in 25 patients of whom 21 were successfully supported with CPB. Patients included in the study were either in cardiac arrest or immediately postarrest with poor systemic perfusion. Only 5 of the 25 patients (20%) included in the analysis sustained a cardiac arrest either in the prehospital or ED setting. Extracorporeal circulation was established by placing a drainage cannula in a central vein, most commonly the femoral, and the infusion cannula in a central artery, most commonly the femoral. After extracorporeal circulation was initiated, patients were treated with an aggressive hemodynamic optimization strategy, transfusing packed red blood cells to maintain a hematocrit of 40%, maximizing ECPR flow (~ 5 L/min) to minimize native cardiac work, and infusing sodium bicarbonate to maintain a minimum arterial pH of 7.30. In addition, lung rest was instituted using pressure control ventilation at a rate of 6 breaths per minute, and initial postarrest volume overload was treated with IV furosemide to maintain a urine output of at least 100 mL/hour. Survivors were on ECPR support for a shorter time than nonsurvivors (44 ± 21 hours vs 87 ± 96 hours; P = .21). Seven of the 9 patients who achieved ROSC survived to hospital discharge. All but one (an end-stage cardiomyopathy patient who received heart transplantation) had an arrest of pulmonary cause. Two other patients were transitioned to a left ventricular assist device and were awaiting transplant at the time of publication. Overall survival was 36%, with the majority neurologically intact.

In 2000, Nagao and colleagues[11] from Tokyo published results of a prospective investigation of an alternative CPR strategy, which they dubbed *cardiopulmonary cerebral resuscitation*, combining ECPB with coronary reperfusion strategies and TH. Of the 50 patients treated, 36 were placed on ECPB. Inclusion criteria were age 18 to 74, OHCA with presumed cardiac cause, initial rhythm of VF, and coma on ED arrival. If ROSC could not be achieved shortly after ED arrival, placement of percutaneous ECPB cannulae and an intra-aortic balloon pump was attempted. After successful cannulation, cardiac catheterization was performed. Of the 36 patients placed on ECPB, 4 (11%) never achieved ROSC, and 23 (64%) never achieved adequate blood pressure to maintain native hemodynamics. The remaining 9 (25%) received extended postarrest care, including TH to 34°C for at least 48 hours. Overall survival in the cohort of 50 patients was 30% (15 of 50) with good neurologic outcomes in 24% (12 of 50); for patients treated with TH, survival was 65% (15 of 23), and good neurologic outcomes were achieved in 52% (12 of 23). Unfortunately, survival results for the patients placed on ECPB were not reported separately, and these data cannot be interpreted regarding the efficacy of this alternative resuscitation strategy.

In 2006, Athanasuleas and colleagues,[65] a group of cardiothoracic surgeons, published a 9-year 34-patient convenience sample of cardiac arrest patients treated with an aggressive resuscitation strategy attempting to direct the scope of resuscitation to the heart and brain. This strategy was accomplished by applying three key interventions: (1) monitored CPR and blood pressure treatment to maintain a peak systolic blood pressure of at least 60 mmHg during resuscitation, (2) rapid transition to CPB, and (3) controlled coronary revascularization using amino acid-enhanced warm blood cardioplegia. The majority of these patients (20 of 36; 56%) arrested while having acute myocardial infarction: 3 of them arrested prior to arrival in the cardiac catheterization lab; the other 17 after undergoing percutaneous coronary interventions. The remaining 14 patients arrested in the context of cardiac surgery, most commonly in the ICU after coronary artery bypass graft (CABG) surgery. CPB was instituted in the operating room via a median sternotomy approach in the vast majority of patients (30 of 34; 88%). Warm blood cardioplegia reperfusate included potassium, THAM, dextrose, glutamate, and aspartate; was mixed in a blood-to-reperfusate ratio of 4:1; and was infused at 125 mL/min for 20 minutes. The length of cardiac arrest in this cohort of patients was prolonged, averaging 72 ± 43 minutes, and transfer to the operating room for CPB was delayed in some cases until invasive monitoring demonstrated adequate blood pressure to maintain cerebral perfusion. Regardless of whether CABG was performed, the aorta was cross-clamped during warm blood cardioplegia and the period of CPB was brief, being continued for 30 minutes after the aortic cross-clamp was discontinued. Survival in this select patient population was 74% (27 of 34), and all but 2 survivors were grossly neurologically intact. The investigators contrasted their impressive neurologically intact survival with the lack of survival seen in Martin and colleagues'[63] case series as well as in another series of 29 patients with no survivors.[62] The investigators suggest that ECPB must be part of an integrated strategy to preserve brain function before, during, and after correction of the pathologic condition precipitating the arrest.

The same year, Sung and colleagues[66] from Seoul, South Korea, reported their experience with implementation of emergency PCPS in 22 patients with refractory cardiac arrest. Because of hospital limitations on PCPS expertise, the investigators chose a portable self-priming PCPS system (Capiox emergency bypass system; Terumo, Inc, Tokyo, Japan). Only one of the 22 patients was started on bypass in the ED; the rest had ECPB initiated in the ICU, catheterization lab, or operating room. The mean duration of PCPS was 52 ± 48 hours in the 13 patients (59%) who could be weaned from PCPS. Twelve patients had interventions to correct the cause of arrest including 4 percutaneous coronary interventions and 2 CABGs. Ten of these patients (83%) were able to be weaned from PCPS. Ten patients (44%) survived, all but one neurologically intact. The investigators argue that their success is directly related to the simplicity and rapid deployment of the PCPS combined with an aggressive search for reversible causes of arrest.

In 2008, Chen and colleagues[67] from Taipei, Taiwan, published results of the use of ECPB for refractory in-hospital arrests. Inclusion criteria were 18 to 75 years old, cardiac cause of in-hospital arrest, and CPR duration less than 10 minutes. The extracorporeal CPB equipment had a heparin-coated circuit, centrifugal pump, and hollow-fiber oxygenator (Medtronic, Anaheim, CA, USA). Patients treated with ECPB were compared with patients during the same period who met inclusion criteria but were not treated with ECPB. The decision to initiate ECPB was made by the attending physician. A total of 113 conventional CPR and 59 ECPR patients were enrolled. A one-to-one matching was performed using propensity analysis to control for potential unbalanced covariates. These covariates included age, sex, initial arrest rhythm, time of day of arrest, and comorbidities. The ECPR group was more likely to have interventions directed at reversing the cause of arrest including percutaneous coronary interventions, CABG, and heart transplantation. One-year survival was higher in the ECPR than the conventional CPR group (18.8 vs 9.7%; $P = .007$), and this survival was maintained in the propensity-matched comparison (19.6 vs 13.0%; $P = .006$).

In 2010, Nagao and colleagues[68] published the results of 10 more years of implementation of ECPB for refractory arrest. Between November 2000 and December 2007, 171 met inclusion criteria for this implementation study: witnessed, out-of-hospital cardiac arrest with less than 15 minutes from collapse to paramedic arrival; between 18 and 74 years old; presumed cardiac cause of arrest; defibrillation by either bystander use of an AED or by EMS; and persistent cardiac arrest on ED arrival. Conventional CPR was continued while the attending physician assessed whether the patient met the inclusion criteria for ECPB. Bypass was initiated by Seldinger technique, placing an outflow cannula in the femoral vein and a return cannula in the femoral artery. The CPB system included a centrifugal pump, a hollow-core oxygenator, and a heat exchanger. An intra-aortic balloon pump was also placed, and after pulsatile bypass was instituted, emergent coronary angiography was performed and culprit lesions treated with stent deployment. In addition, hemodynamics were optimized to a MAP of 90 to 120 mmHg and a pulmonary artery occlusion pressure of 15 to 20mmHg. Mild TH was instituted as soon as possible after the patient was on functional CPB with a target temperature of 34°C, which was maintained for 3 days after target temperature was reached (**Fig. 3**). Using this approach, 19.3% of the patients (44 of 171) survived to hospital discharge, and 12.3% (21 of 171) survived with favorable neurologic outcomes, defined as Glasgow-Pittsburgh Cerebral Performance score of 1 or 2.

A recent report from Japan is the first to attempt to compare the effectiveness of ECPB for refractory cardiac arrest versus standard ALS.[69] The SAVE-J consortium

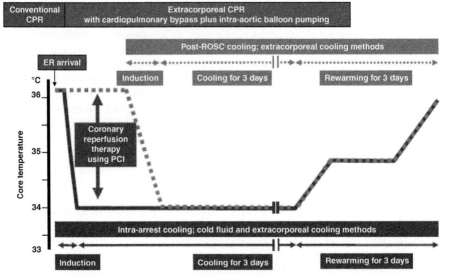

Fig. 3. Protocol of ECPR for induction of hypothermia with percutaneous coronary intervention (PCI). After arrival at the emergency room, ECPR using emergency cardiopulmonary bypass plus intra-aortic balloon pumping was immediately performed. Subsequently, emergency coronary angiography with PCI was performed in cases of suspected acute coronary syndrome. The goal was to reach a target temperature of 34°C within 6 hours in the post-ROSC cooling group (*upper dotted part and dotted line*), and within 30 minutes in the intraarrest cooling group (*lower gray part and gray line*). (*From* Nagao K, Kikushima K, Watanabe K, et al. Early induction of hypothermia during cardiac arrest improves neurologic outcomes in patients with out-of-hospital cardiac arrest who undergo emergency cardiopulmonary bypass and percutaneous coronary intervention. Circ J 2010;74:77–85; with permission.)

consisted of 46 participating EDs, with 26 using a protocolized ECPB strategy for refractory arrest and 20 departments using standard ALS care. All hospitals used standardized ALS for the initial 15 minutes of cardiac arrest treatment and included TH and hemodynamic optimization in their postarrest management protocol. At the ECPB hospitals, ECPB was performed on eligible patients who were observed at some point to have a rhythm of VF, were under 75 years old, required less than 45 minutes from collapse to the ED, and who remained pulseless after 15 minutes of full ED ALS efforts. With standard ACLS and protocolized postarrest care centered on TH, there were 2 survivors (1.6%) with good neurologic function at 30 days out of 134 patients treated, whereas with ECPB there were 22 survivors out of 183 patients treated (12%). This study is ongoing, but the large difference in survival is the first attempt to directly compare ECPB versus standard ALS care.

SUMMARY

ECPB is a relatively new, advanced resuscitation method that is growing in technical sophistication, shows promising experimental data, and is expanding in clinical practice. Experimental data and clinical studies suggest its ability to be highly effective at producing ROSC for refractory cardiac arrest. Currently however, the majority of patients who achieve ROSC with ECPB do not survive long-term with good neurologic function. Despite this limitation, survival rates may be far better than standard ALS care.

Nichol and colleagues[70] performed a systematic review of PCPS for cardiac arrest and refractory shock and identified 85 studies with a total of 1494 treated with PCPS for refractory shock or cardiac arrest. Overall survival was 47.4%. When limited to PCPS used to treat cardiac arrest, the investigators found 54 studies with 674 patients, 44.9% of whom survived to discharge. In funnel plot analyses of survival versus sample size for cardiogenic shock and cardiac arrest patients, they found that the plots were skewed to the left—with higher survival in publications with fewer patients. This result suggests publication bias, as is typical of early technologies. The investigators concluded that their review demonstrated that PCPS is an efficacious intervention in cardiogenic shock and cardiac arrest. However, they acknowledged that "high-quality, adequately controlled trials are required to determine whether percutaneous bypass is effective." In preparation for the 2010 AHA CPR guidelines, members of the International Liaison Committee on Resuscitation reviewed the data for efficacy of ECPB to treat refractory arrest. They recommended that a "further prospective control trial for out-of-hospital cardiac arrest with long-term follow-up is desired to clarify . . . [the] effectiveness of . . . extracorporeal cardiopulmonary support."[71]

THE FUTURE

The future of ECPB will depend on new data gathered in the next decade. There are significant opportunities and methodologies that may be further optimized to improve survival using ECPB. The collective data on ECPB suggest that it may be the best hope available for survival in patients with refractory cardiac arrest.

REFERENCES

1. Travers AH, Rea TD, Bobrow BJ, et al. CPR Overview: 2010 American Heart Association Guidelines for Cardiopulmonary Resuscitation and Emergency Cardiovascular Care. Circulation 2010;122:S676–84.
2. Peberdy MA, Kaye W, Ornato JP, et al. Cardiopulmonary resuscitation of adults in the hospital: a report of 14720 cardiac arrests from the National Registry of Cardiopulmonary Resuscitation. Resuscitation 2003;58:297–308.
3. Weisfeldt ML, Becker LB. Resuscitation after cardiac arrest: a 3-phase time-sensitive model [comment]. JAMA 2002;288:3035–8.
4. Cummins R, Eisenberg MS, Hallstrom A, et al. Survival of out-of-hospital cardiac arrest with early initiation of cardiopulmonary resuscitation. Am J Emerg Med 1985; 3:114–8.
5. Pionkowski R, Thompson B, Gruchow J, et al. Resuscitation time in ventricular fibrillation a prognostic indicator. Ann Emerg Med 1984;12:733–8.
6. Laurent I, Adrie C, Vinsonneau C, et al. High-volume hemofiltration after out-of-hospital cardiac arrest: a randomized study. J Am Coll Cardiol 2005;46:432–7.
7. Stammers A. Historical aspects of cardiopulmonary bypass: from antiquity to acceptance. J Cardiothorac Vasc Anesth 1997;11:266–74.
8. Gibbon J. Artificial maintenance of circulation during experimental occlusion of the pulmonary artery. Arch Surg 1937;34:1105–37.
9. Follette D, Steed D, Foglia R, et al. Reduction of postischemic myocardial damage by maintaining arrest during initial reperfusion. Surg Forum 1977;28:281–3.
10. Follette D, Fey K, Steed D, et al. Reducing reperfusion injury with hypocalcemic, hyperkalemic, alkalotic blood during reoxygenation. Surg Forum 1978;29:284–6.
11. Nagao K, Hayashi N, Kanmatsuse K, et al. Cardiopulmonary cerebral resuscitation using emergency cardiopulmonary bypass, coronary reperfusion therapy and mild hypothermia in patients with cardiac arrest outside the hospital. J Am Coll Cardiol 2000;36:776–83.

12. Ballaux PK, Gourlay T, Ratnatunga CP, et al. A literature review of cardiopulmonary bypass models for rats. Perfusion 1999;14:411–7.
13. Safar P, Abramson NS, Angelos M, et al. Emergency cardiopulmonary bypass for resuscitation from prolonged cardiac arrest. Am J Emerg Med 1990;8:55–67.
14. Reich H, Angelos M, Safar P, et al. Cardiac resuscitability with cardiopulmonary bypass after increasing ventricular fibrillation times in dogs. Ann Emerg Med 1990; 19:887–90.
15. Levine R, Gorayeb M, Safar P, et al. Cardiopulmonary bypass after cardiac arrest and prolonged closed-chest CPR in dogs. Ann Emerg Med 1987;16:620–7.
16. Angelos M, Safar P, Reich H. A comparison of cardiopulmonary resuscitation with cardiopulmonary bypass after prolonged cardiac arrest in dogs. Reperfusion pressures and neurologic recovery. Resuscitation 1991;21:121–35.
17. Ao H, Tanimoto H, Yoshitake A, et al. Long-term mild hypothermia with extracorporeal lung and heart assist improves survival from prolonged cardiac arrest in dogs. Resuscitation 2001;48:163–74.
18. Tanimoto H, Ichinose K, Okamoto T, et al. Rapidly induced hypothermia with extracorporeal lung and heart assist (ECLHA) improves the neurological outcome after prolonged cardiac arrest in dogs. Resuscitation 2007;72:128–36.
19. Safar P, Xiao F, Radovsky A, et al. Improved cerebral resuscitation from cardiac arrest in dogs with mild hypothermia plus blood flow promotion. Stroke 1996;27:105–13.
20. Han F, Boller M, Guo W, et al. A rodent model of emergency cardiopulmonary bypass resuscitation with different temperatures after asphyxial cardiac arrest. Resuscitation 2010;81:83–99.
21. Nozari A, Safar P, Stezoski SW, et al. Critical time window for intra-arrest cooling with cold saline flush in a dog model of cardiopulmonary resuscitation. Circulation 2006; 113:2690–6.
22. Behringer W, Kentner R, Wu X, et al. Fructose-1,6-bisphosphate and MK-801 by aortic arch flush for cerebral preservation during exsanguination cardiac arrest of 20 min in dogs. An exploratory study. Resuscitation 2001;50:205–16.
23. Behringer W, Prueckner S, Kentner R, et al. Rapid hypothermic aortic flush can achieve survival without brain damage after 30 minutes cardiac arrest in dogs. Anesthesiology 2000;93:1491–9.
24. Behringer W, Prueckner S, Safar P, et al. Rapid induction of mild cerebral hypothermia by cold aortic flush achieves normal recovery in a dog outcome model with 20-minute exsanguination cardiac arrest. Acad Emerg Med 2000;7:1341–8.
25. Behringer W, Safar P, Wu X, et al. Survival without brain damage after clinical death of 60-120 mins in dogs using suspended animation by profound hypothermia. Crit Care Med 2003;31:1523–31.
26. Safar P, Tisherman SA, Behringer W, et al. Suspended animation for delayed resuscitation from prolonged cardiac arrest that is unresuscitable by standard cardiopulmonary-cerebral resuscitation. Crit Care Med 2000;28:N214–8.
27. Sterz F, Leonov Y, Safar P, et al. Hypertension with or without hemodilution after cardiac arrest in dogs. Stroke 1990;21:1178–84.
28. Sanderson JM, Wright G, Sims FW. Brain damage in dogs immediately following pulsatile and non-pulsatile blood flows in extracorporeal circulation. Thorax 1972;27: 275–86.
29. Wright G, Sanderson JM. Brain damage and mortality in dogs following pulsatile and non-pulsatile blood flows in extracorporeal circulation. Thorax 1972;27:738–49.
30. Taylor KM, Devlin BJ, Mittra SM, et al. Assessment of cerebral damage during open-heart surgery. A new experimental model. Scand J Thorac Cardiovasc Surg 1980;14:197–203.

31. Onoe M, Mori A, Watarida S, et al. The effect of pulsatile perfusion on cerebral blood flow during profound hypothermia with total circulatory arrest. J Thorac Cardiovasc Surg 1994;108:119–25.
32. Ohnishi Y, Hu Q-H, Yamaguchi S, et al. Cerebral microcirculatory changes in rat with a cardiopulmonary bypass using fluorescence videomicroscopy. Clin Hemorheol Microcirc 2002;26:15–26.
33. Briceno JC, Runge TM. Monitoring of blood gases during prolonged experimental cardiopulmonary bypass and their relationship to brain pH, PO2, and PCO2. ASAIO J 1994;40:M344–50.
34. Mori Y, Ueno K, Hattori A, et al. Emergency cardiopulmonary bypass support in patients with cardiac arrest caused by myocardial infarction. Artif Organs 1994;18:698–701.
35. Sezai A, Shiono M, Nakata K-I, et al. Effects of pulsatile CPB on interleukin-8 and endothelin-1 levels. Artif Organs 2005;29:708–13.
36. Anstadt MP, Stonnington MJ, Tedder M, et al. Pulsatile reperfusion after cardiac arrest improves neurologic outcome. Ann Surg 1991;214:478–88.
37. Liakopoulos OJ, Hristov N, Buckberg GD, et al. Resuscitation after prolonged cardiac arrest: effects of cardiopulmonary bypass and sodium-hydrogen exchange inhibition on myocardial and neurological recovery. Eur J Cardiothorac Surg 2011;40:978–84.
38. Trummer G, Foerster K, Buckberg GD, et al. Successful resuscitation after prolonged periods of cardiac arrest: a new field in cardiac surgery. J Thorac Cardiovasc Surg 2010;139:1325–32.
39. Meloni BP, Campbell K, Zhu H, et al. In search of clinical neuroprotection after brain ischemia. Stroke 2009;40:2236–40.
40. Katz LM, Wang Y, Rockoff S, et al. Low-dose Carbicarb improves cerebral outcome after asphyxial cardiac arrest in rats. Ann Emerg Med 2002;39:359–65.
41. Cohen MV, Yang X-M, Downey JM. The pH hypothesis of postconditioning: staccato reperfusion reintroduces oxygen and perpetuates myocardial acidosis. Circulation 2007;115:1895–903.
42. Inserte J, Barba I, Hernando V, et al. Delayed recovery of intracellular acidosis during reperfusion prevents calpain activation and determines protection in postconditioned myocardium. Cardiovasc Res 2009;81:116–22.
43. Hirleman E, Larson DF. Cardiopulmonary bypass and edema: physiology and pathophysiology. Perfusion 2008;23:311–22.
44. Bottiger BW, Motsch J, Braun V, et al. Marked activation of complement and leukocytes and an increase in the concentrations of soluble endothelial adhesion molecules during cardiopulmonary resuscitation and early reperfusion after cardiac arrest in humans. Crit Care Med 2002;30:2473–80.
45. Levy JH, Tanaka KA. Inflammatory response to cardiopulmonary bypass. Ann Thorac Surg 2003;75:S715–20.
46. Rinder CS, Bonan JL, Rinder HM, et al. Cardiopulmonary bypass induces leukocyte-platelet adhesion. Blood 1992;79:1201–5.
47. Allen BS, Castella M, Buckberg GD, et al. Conditioned blood reperfusion markedly enhances neurologic recovery after prolonged cerebral ischemia. J Thorac Cardiovasc Surg 2003;126:1851–8.
48. Allen BS, Veluz JS, Buckberg GD, et al. Deep hypothermic circulatory arrest and global reperfusion injury: avoidance by making a pump prime reperfusate a new concept. J Thorac Cardiovasc Surg 2003;125:625–32.
49. Bolling KS, Halldorsson A, Allen BS, et al. Prevention of the hypoxic reoxygenation injury with the use of a leukocyte-depleting filter. J Thorac Cardiovasc Surg 1997;113:1081–9.

50. Kilgannon JH, Jones AE, Parrillo JE, et al. Relationship between supranormal oxygen tension and outcome after resuscitation from cardiac arrest. Circulation 2011;123: 2717–22.

51. Idris AH, Roberts LJ 2nd, Caruso L, et al. Oxidant injury occurs rapidly after cardiac arrest, cardiopulmonary resuscitation, and reperfusion. Crit Care Med 2005;33: 2043–8.

52. Balan IS, Fiskum G, Hazelton J, et al. Oximetry-guided reoxygenation improves neurological outcome after experimental cardiac arrest. Stroke 2006;37: 3008–13.

53. Yoshitake A, Tanimoto H, Ao H, et al. Does veno-arterial bypass without an artificial lung improve the outcome in dogs undergoing cardiac arrest? Resuscitation 2002; 54:159–66.

54. Wenzel V, Padosch SA, Voelckel WG, et al. Survey of effects of anesthesia protocols on hemodynamic variables in porcine cardiopulmonary resuscitation laboratory models before induction of cardiac arrest. Comp Med 2000;50:644–8.

55. Papadimitriou D, Xanthos T, Dontas I, et al. The use of mice and rats as animal models for cardiopulmonary resuscitation research. Lab Anim 2008;42:265–76.

56. van der Worp HB, Howells DW, Sena ES, et al. Can animal models of disease reliably inform human studies? PLoS Med 2010;7:e1000245.

57. Engdahl J, Holmberg M, Karlson BW, et al. The epidemiology of out-of-hospital 'sudden' cardiac arrest. Resuscitation 2002;52:235–45.

58. Wang L, Traystman RJ, Murphy SJ, et al. Inhalational anesthetics as preconditioning agents in ischemic brain. Curr Opin Pharmacol 2008;8:104–10.

59. Ichinose K, Okamoto T, Tashiro M, et al. The effects of pre-arrest heparin administration dose for cardiac arrest model using extracorporeal lung and a heart assist (ECLHA) in dogs. Resuscitation 2006;69:311–8.

60. Mattox K, Beall AJ. Resuscitation of the moribund patient using portable cardiopulmonary bypass. Ann Thorac Surg 1976;22:436–42.

61. Reichman RT, Joyo CI, Dembitsky WP, et al. Improved patient survival after cardiac arrest using a cardiopulmonary support system. Ann Thorac Surg 1990; 49:101–4.

62. Hartz R, LoCicero J 3rd, Sanders JH Jr, et al. Clinical experience with portable cardiopulmonary bypass in cardiac arrest patients. Ann Thorac Surg 1990;50: 437–41.

63. Martin GB, Rivers EP, Paradis NA, et al. Emergency department cardiopulmonary bypass in the treatment of human cardiac arrest. Chest 1998;113:743–51.

64. Younger JG, Schreiner RJ, Swaniker F, et al. Extracorporeal resuscitation of cardiac arrest. Acad Emerg Med 1999;6:700–7.

65. Athanasuleas C, Buckberg G, Allen B, et al. Sudden cardiac death: directing the scope of resuscitation towards the heart and brain. Resuscitation 2006;70:44–51.

66. Sung K, Lee Y, Park P, et al. Improved survival after cardiac arrest using emergent autopriming percutaneous cardiopulmonary support. Ann Thorac Surg 2006;82: 651–6.

67. Chen Y, Lin J, Yu H, et al. Cardiopulmonary resuscitation with assisted extracorporeal life-support versus conventional cardiopulmonary resuscitation in adults with in-hospital cardiac arrest: an observational study and propensity analysis. Lancet 2008;372:554–61.

68. Nagao K, Kikushima K, Watanabe K, et al. Early induction of hypothermia during cardiac arrest improves neurologic outcomes in patients with out-of-hospital cardiac arrest who undergo emergency cardiopulmonary bypass and percutaneous coronary intervention. Circ J 2010;74:77–85.

69. Sakamoto T, Asai Y, Nagao K, et al. Multicenter non-randomized prospective cohort study of extracorporeal cardiopulmonary resuscitation for out-of hospital cardiac arrest: Study of Advanced Life Support for Ventricular Fibrillation with Extracorporeal Circulation in Japan (SAVE-J). Circulation 2011;124:A18132.
70. Nichol G, Karmy-Jones R, Salerno C, et al. Systematic review of percutaneous cardiopulmonary bypass for cardiac arrest or cardiogenic shock states. Resuscitation 2006;70:381–94.
71. ILCOR Worksheet. Available at: http://circ.ahajournals.org/site/C2010/ALS-CPR-A-002A.pdf. Accessed November 23, 2011.

Therapeutic Hypothermia After Cardiac Arrest in Adults: Mechanism of Neuroprotection, Phases of Hypothermia, and Methods of Cooling

Yinlun Weng, MD[a], Shijie Sun, MD[a,b],*

KEYWORDS

- Cardiac arrest • Cardiopulmonary resuscitation
- Hypothermia • Neurologic function

Sudden cardiac arrest is the main manifestation of ischemic heart diseases, which is the leading cause of death worldwide. Each year an estimated 300,000 people suffer from cardiac arrest in the United States, with a variable incidence ranging from 36/100,000 to 128/100,000.[1–4] Approximately 7.9% of cardiac arrest victims survive to hospital discharge in the United States,[5] whereas fewer than half of patients admitted to hospital achieve a favorable outcome. Permanent severe brain damage accounts for the high mortality after successful resuscitation in the hospital.

Mild hypothermia, defined here as a reduction of core temperature to 32°C to 34°C, is the only proven therapy to improve survival and neurologic outcome after sudden cardiac arrest in clinical trials, and recommended by the American Heart Association (AHA) as the routine intervention for selected comatose adult victims of witnessed out-of-hospital cardiac arrest.[6–10] This article addresses the mechanism of neuroprotection, phases of hypothermia, and cooling methods.

The authors have received financial support through an American Heart Association grant (11IRG 487001). The authors have no relationship with any commercial company that has a direct financial interest in the subject matter or materials discussed in their article or with a company making a competing product.

a The Weil Institute of Critical Care Medicine, 35100 Bob Hope Drive, Rancho Mirage, CA 92270, USA
b Keck School of Medicine of the University of Southern California, Health Sciences Campus, Los Angeles, CA 90089, USA
* Corresponding author. The Weil Institute of Critical Care Medicine, 35100 Bob Hope Drive, Rancho Mirage, CA 92270.
E-mail address: shijiesun@aol.com

Crit Care Clin 28 (2012) 231–243
doi:10.1016/j.ccc.2011.10.012
0749-0704/12/$ – see front matter © 2012 Elsevier Inc. All rights reserved.

MECHANISMS OF NEUROPROTECTION

In recent years, there has been significant progress in our understanding of cerebral injury after cardiac arrest. There are three phases in cerebral injury after hypoxic insult: early, intermediate, and late. In the early stage, absence of cerebral blood flow occurs immediately after cardiac arrest despite ongoing consumption of oxygen, adenosine triphosphate, and glucose.[11–14] In the intermediate phase, release of excitatory amino acids and glutamate in the brain activates destructive cytotoxic cascades such as free radicals and nitric oxide hours after the arrest.[12] In the late phase, a series of injuries may occur up to 24 hours after cardiac arrest, including breakdown of the blood–brain barrier, exacerbation of cerebral edema, and neuronal death.[11,12] Therapeutic hypothermia might exert neuroprotection by multiple mechanisms in the single or synergistic aforementioned phases, including reduction of brain metabolism, attenuation of reactive oxygen species formation, inhibition of excitatory amino acid release, attenuation of the immune response during reperfusion. and blockage of apoptosis.

Reduction of Brain Metabolism

Hypothermia produced a decrease of cerebral metabolism by 6% to 10% per 1°C reduction in core body temperature, reflected by decreases in energy utilization and consumption of oxygen and glucose.[15–30] This mechanism was not the only explanation for the dramatic difference seen despite the certain role of metabolic decrease in neuroprotection.[31]

Attenuation of Neuroexcitotoxic Cascade

Depletion of ATP after hypoxia results in intracellular and extracellular acidosis, failure of ATP-dependent Na^+,K^+-ATPase, imbalance of the cellular Na^+ gradient, and Ca^{2+} influx into neurons. This would further lead to cellular depolarization that causes a release of excitatory amino acids such as glutamate. In turn, it further promotes Ca^{2+} influx. Because of the characteristic of ATP or oxygen dependence, the Ca^{2+} sequestration ultimately collapses, leading to loss of the calcium-buffering capacity. Hypothermia has been proved to potentially attenuate the aforementioned steps of neuroexcitotoxic cascade that causes cell death.[32–34]

Abolition of Reactive Oxygen Species

Another important destructive process is the release of reactive oxygen species that followed reperfusion of oxygenated blood after cardiac arrest. Reactive oxygen species could directly damage numerous cellular components such as neuronal lipid membranes, proteins, and DNA through peroxidation.[35] Even if neurons possess various enzymatic and nonenzymatic antioxidant mechanisms that prevent peroxidative injury, these intrinsic effects are overwhelmed by the production of free radical production after ischemia–reperfusion. Antioxidant depletion and byproducts of peroxidation have shown to peak up to 16 hours after restoration of circulation, suggesting that neuronal injury continues long after the initial resuscitation.[36,37] Hypothermia significantly decreased the quantity of free radicals, which would reserve more space or time for endogenous protective mechanisms in counteracting the oxidative damage.[38–41]

Inhibition of Apoptosis

Cells suffering from ischemia and reperfusion face three fates: necrosis, apoptosis, or full or partial recovery. The initiating and determinant factor for induction of apoptosis is the interaction of proapoptotic and antiapoptotic factors; it is influenced by the disturbed energy metabolism, dysfunctional mitochondria, and the release of caspase enzymes. Hypothermia appears to affect these processes in different ways. In the presence of hypothermia, the antiapoptosis protein Bcl-2 is enhanced whereas proapoptosis BAX is suppressed. Hypothermia would interfere with depletion of energy metabolism, which would lead to overload of calcium and release of glutamate and contribute to the induction of apoptosis. Hypothermia to some extent attenuated the mitochondrial dysfunction by inhibition of translocation of cytochrome *c* into cytosol.[42] Inactivation of caspase enzyme would further contribute to the prevention of apoptosis by hypothermia.[42–45] In addition, apoptosis occurs relatively late in the postperfusion phase and lasts for 48 to 72 hours or even longer, providing a wide window of opportunity for intervention.[45–47]

Suppression of the Inflammatory Response

The inflammatory response in most types of ischemia cerebral injury is mediated by proinflammatory mediators such tumor necrosis factor-α (TNF-α); interleukin (IL)-1, -2, -10; macrophage inflammatory protein-1α; and growth-related oncogene/KC.[48] The chemotaxis of activated leukocytes across the blood–brain barrier is then stimulated, leading to accumulation of inflammatory cells in the injured brain and expression of adhesion molecules on leukocytes and endothelial cells, while the passage of neutrophils and monocytes–macrophages is activated by the complement systems. The inflammatory response begins and peaks within 1 hour and lasts for up to 5 days.[49] Because the inflammatory response may be physiologic, the extent of cytokine production and leukocyte infiltration would then determine if the physiologic response would not be overwhelmed by the destructive aspects of inflammation.[49–51] Hypothermia has been proved to effectively suppress the ischemia- evoked inflammatory response by inhibiting neutrophil infiltration, reducing lipid peroxidation and leukotriene production, and decreasing the overexpression of nitric oxide.[32,52–54]

Protection of Blood–Brain Barrier Integrity

Blood–brain barrier integrity was destroyed after ischemia and reperfusion after cardiac arrest through decreased fluidity and integrity of cell membranes and increased vascular permeability of microvascular endothelial cells in the brain.[55,56] The entire process was mediated by vascular endothelial growth factors via release of nitric oxide. The disruption of the blood–brain barrier would further contribute to exacerbation of brain edema. Hypothermia significantly prevents the progressive development of vascular permeability and the resultant formation of edema after ischemia reperfusion.[57–59]

TEMPERATURE PHASES IN HYPOTHERMIA

Temperature modulation during therapeutic hypothermia occurs in three phases: induction, maintenance, and rewarming.

Induction Phase

Optimal variables, such as onset of cooling, target temperature, and the rate of cooling to the target temperature remain unclear. In the setting of cardiac arrest, there are numerous data supporting the importance of early initiation of hypothermia as soon as possible after restoration of spontaneous circulation (ROSC); in animal models, efficiency is enhanced when hypothermia is initiated before arrest or coincident with the arrest.[60–64] More data prove that with the delay of implementation of hypothermia, the beneficial effects of hypothermia were negated in overall performance, neurologic deficit, and brain histopathologic damage.[65–68] It is unrealistic for sudden cardiac death to induce therapeutic hypothermia before cardiac arrest except accidental hypothermia. There is no human study indicating the time from initiation of therapy to achieve therapeutic temperature is a significant predictor of outcome, and the optimal rate of cooling is unknown. Notably, immediate side effects such as hypovolemia, electrolyte disorders, and hyperglycemia occur in the induction period, representing the greatest patient management problems.[69–71] In this sense, to reduce the risk, it would be more appropriate to provide a rapid induction of hypothermia, including shortening the duration of the induction phase and reaching the more stable maintenance phase as quickly as possible. With respect to the target temperature, it is recommended to cool down to 32°C to 34°C based on the American Heart Association (AHA) guideline[8]; however, Gal and colleagues proved that therapeutic hypothermia with the target temperature of 34°C to 35°C was more easily attainable, feasible, safe, and efficient in patients after cardiac arrest and with fewer side effects.[72] A significantly decreased rate of refibrillation and need for late defibrillation was found when the milder hypothermia of 35°C was applied.[73]

Maintenance Phase

In this phase, there are two marked issues: the duration of hypothermia and stability in controlling the core temperature. Although the 2010 AHA guideline recommended providing duration of 12 to 24 hours of hypothermia, there are different viewpoints. Dietrich and colleagues[74] demonstrated that hypothermia of 30°C for 3 hours after global brain ischemia produced short-term protection (3 and 7 days postischemia) but not long-lasting protection (6 months), which was reported to be present in extended hypothermia of 32°C from 12 to 24 hours in gerbils and 32°C to 34°C for 48 hours in rats in the studies by Colbourne and Corbett.[75,76] Hickey and colleagues[77] demonstrated that even spontaneously hypothermia, which initiated within several hours and recovered to nomothermia within 24 to 36 hours, still had a neuroprotective effect. Recently the study in a rat model of 2 hours of occlusion of the middle cerebral artery (MCAO) by Shintani and colleagues[78] identified that mild hypothermia at 35°C should be introduced within 4 hours after MCAO and maintained for longer than 4 hours to achieve neuroprotective effects. Conversely, Agnew and colleagues reported a prolonged effect without negative side effects using a prolonged (>24 hours) cooling period in asphyxic cardiac arrest piglet models.[79] It also has been proved that a longer duration of cooling should decrease the volume of infarction of after cerebral artery occlusion.[80] The discordance between these studies suggests that the window and duration of hypothermia depend on the animal model, the severity of the injury, and even the paradigm of hypothermia. As to the stability, it would be better to control core temperature tightly with minor or no fluctuation (maximum 0.2°C–0.5°C).[81] With a lower incidence of shivering response, hypovolemia, and electrolyte loss in the maintenance phase, attention should be shifted toward the long-term side effects such as nosocomial infections and bedsores.

Rewarming Phase

There is still controversy regarding the rewarming rate. In general, the successful protection provided via hypothermia intervention is associated with a relatively slow course of posthypothermia rewarming. Bernard and coworkers found 1.0°C per 1.4 hours of rewarming has no adverse hemodynamic effects.[7] The HACA study group indicated that passive rewarming with a rate of 1.0°C every 2 hours did not counteract the effect of hypothermia.[6] Busch demonstrated that a rewarming rate of 1.0°C every

2.5 hours benefits the outcome, accompanied with an occasional rebound hypothermia.[82] In contrast, when most animal studies were replicated with more rapid rewarming, not only were the beneficial effects of hypothermia eliminated, but in most cases, the ensuing pathology also was markedly exacerbated.[83,84] In terms of the mechanistic perspective, the damaging consequences of rapid rewarming are not yet fully understood; numerous evidence suggests injury resulting from rapid rewarming was related to exacerbation of mitochondrial permeability transition and enhanced generation of oxygen free radicals.[83,85] First, rapid rewarming could cause electrolyte disorders caused by shifts from the intracellular to the extracellular compartment. Second, insulin sensitivity could increase during rewarming. Third, rapid rewarming could lead to loss of some or even all of the protective effects of hypothermia.[86–90]

COOLING METHODS

An ideal cooling method is expected to be characterized by the following features: rapid cooling, homogeneous cooling, cost effectiveness, easy implementation, portability, safety, and effective control. A growing number of cooling methods are emerging, which could be simply classified as noninvasive surface cooling and invasive cooling. Surface cooling devices are noninvasive and range from simple ice packs to sophisticated machines with automatic feedback controls. Invasive cooling methods include the administration of ice-cold fluids intravenously, intravascular cooling catheters, body cavity lavage, extracorporeal circuits, and selective brain cooling.

Surface Cooling

Ice packs are considered one of the simplest approaches for inducing hypothermia. It is as simple to apply as just attaching into head, neck, torso, and extremities. Ice packs are reported to provide a relatively slow cooling rate of 0.9°C per hour.[7] Even combined with towels soaked in ice water, it still takes a median of 7.5 hours to achieve mild hypothermia.[91] In addition, the use of alcohol and fans is limited because of safety and hygiene concerns. However, one of the primary limitations of these methods is inferior temperature control. Therefore, it would require more dependence on nursing care to avoid overshoot of cooling and unintentional rewarming.

Some surface devices such as cooling blankets (Arctic Sun, Medivance, Louisville, CO, USA) make it possible to operate with feedback control by circulating water through specially designed pads and conductively exchange heat with skin to achieve a cooling rate of 1.2°C per hour.[91,92] In addition to its servo control, this device is radiolucent to facilitate the imaging study without causing a fluctuation of temperature by removal the device. However, there are some disadvantages of this technique, such as inability to monitor the condition of skin under the blanket and risk of skin sloughing.

Immersion of the body in ice water would be a highly efficient strategy but difficult to control.[93] This approach is adopted by Thermosuit System (Life Recovery Systems, Kinnelon, NJ, USA), which surrounds patients directly with cool water and also possesses a feedback control unit with a safe and effective underwater defibrillation. Animal studies suggest that it provides a cooling rate of 9.7°C per hour in 30-kg pigs, in contrast with 3.0°C per hour in human data.[91,94,95]

EMCOOLSPads (Emcools, Vienna, Austria) is another feasible, safe method. It uses plates of mixed ice and graphite to enhance thermal conductivity, avoiding the low efficiency when water melting on ice cubes inhibits effective cooling with ice alone. In addition, this device is independent of power supply, thus making it especially appropriate for out-of-hospital use. It has been used by emergency medical services (EMS) in 15 patients in a prehospital study with a cooling rate of 3.3°C per hour.[91,96]

Nasopharyngeal evaporative cooling with the Rhino-Chill-device (BeneChill, San Diego, CA, USA) is a novel method that sprays a convective coolant via a catheter in the nasal cavity, thus cooling the basal brain region. It is demonstrated to exert a cooling rate of 2.4 and 1.4°C per hour for tympanic and core temperature, respectively, and seemingly related to improved defibrillation success.[91,97] In addition, this device operates independent of energy source, which makes it appealing for use out of hospital.

Invasive Cooling

The infusion of cold fluids has the advantage of being inexpensive, effective, and easily available. Infusion speed and muscle paralysis are two factors affecting the effectiveness, so that clinically large-gauge cannulas and pressure bags are adopted to increase the speed and muscle paralysis is included to avoid shivering.[91] Berard and colleagues used infusion of cold Ringer's lactate at a rate of 30 mL/kg for 30 minutes in cardiac arrest survivors, and found it could provide a rate of 3.4°C per hour.[98] Notably, no pulmonary edema occurred as a result of the fluid load; instead, a rise in mean artery blood pressure was observed.[98] Another study by Kim and coworkers adopted a protocol of infusion of 2000 mL of ice-cold saline over 30 minutes, demonstrating no effect on electrolyte balance, cardiac function, central venous pressure, pulmonary pressures, and left atrial filling pressure, and even a slight improvement in ejection fraction 1 hour after infusion.[99] Data are available to support that the effectiveness of cold fluids is dependent on choice of fluid, such as saline, lactated Ringer's solution, or others.[98–102] As Kin and coworkers demonstrated, an approximately 1.24°C reduction of temperature was achieved in a 63-patient randomized trial with no adverse effects, supporting that administration of cold saline also proved to be suitable for out-of-hospital use.[103] The use of cold fluids for advanced cardiac life support (ACLS) has been demonstrated in animal and human studies, suggesting that this method also produced a beneficial outcome including achievement of mild hypothermia and improved defibrillation without an adverse effect in the hemodynamic variable of cerebral blood flow.[73,104–107] One disadvantage of infusion of cold fluids is its fluctuation of maintaining the target temperature after induction; only a small percentage of patients did not rewarm spontaneously during observation after induction without other intervention.[91] Based on the compatibility of cold fluids, a combination of other interventions to avoid spontaneous rewarming is recommended, such as a cooling catheter and cooling blanket.

Intravascular devices are designed to exchange heat through a catheter containing circulating saline at a controlled temperature with a feedback of patient temperature. The CoolGard System (Alsius, Irvine, CA, USA) is one of the products adopting this mechanism. This system has been used in patients after resuscitation, yielding a cooling rate of approximately 1.0°C per hour in human studies.[108,109] This method is advantageous in close temperature control for maintenance and rewarming from hypothermia, but disadvantageous in risks of bleeding, vessel thrombosis, and catheter-related infection.

Other Approaches

Recently pharmacologic hypothermia has been considered for its easy implementation. An analogue of neurotensin was reported to induce hypothermia rapidly in rats after intravenous administration in a model of asphyxic cardiac arrest and reduce neurologic injury as compared with external cooling.[110] Sun and colleagues have demonstrated that the nonselective cannabinoid receptors agonist WIN55, 212-2 induced a reduction of 3.2°C in blood temperature within 4 hours and benefited postresuscitation myocardial and neurologic function without compromised hemo-dynamics.[111] Cholesystokinin octapeptide (CCK8) was also proven to induce a decrease of 2.2°C in blood temperature within 4 hours in a rat model of cardiac arrest and resuscitation and produced a significant beneficial effects in postresuscitation myocardial and neurologic function.[112]

Venovenous cooling is a dialysis method using a double-lumen catheter to connect with the femoral vein and an extracorporeal heat exchanger for rapid blood cooling. The method in the pig study allowed for a cooling rate of 8.2°C per hour.[113] However, this method can also be invasive and, with the risks of bleeding and infection, likely no more useful than other less invasive devices.

Total liquid ventilation with perflourcarbon produces effective hypothermia while allowing oxygenation and ventilation; it has been proved in a swine model of cardiopulmonary resuscitation (CPR) to improve the ROSC rate.[114,115]

Ice slurries, smoothed 100-mm ice particles at a subzero temperature, provide another relatively more effective cooling method than conventional cold fluid, with a reduction of 4°C in brain temperature in a pig experiment.[91]

Although many devices are available to achieve therapeutic hypothermia, there are no current data recommending one method over another. All of the factors involving the individual institute and the condition of patients should be taken into consideration when making a decision regarding the optimal method to apply.

SUMMARY

Mild therapeutic hypothermia proved to be the first treatment to reverse postischemic cerebral injury in clinical studies. To maximize the efficiency of cooling, more attention should be focused on understanding the mechanisms underlying its protective effects, the phases involving its management problems, and the methods relevant to its realistic strategy. Inevitably, there are other aspects that are not appreciated or somewhat overestimated, raising the great need for further research and more comprehensive knowledge of therapeutic hypothermia.

From the perspective of neuroprotection, more issues need to be explored such as onset and duration of hypothermia, target temperature, rewarming strategy, and more detailed and feasible protocols in choosing the individual cooling device. Most importantly, avoid discouragement, as even the simplest method, such as ice packs, can be effective.

REFERENCES

1. Galea S, Blaney S, Nandi A, et al. Explaining racial disparities in incidence of and survival from out-of-hospital cardiac arrest. Am J Epidemiol 2007;166(5):534–43.
2. Cobb LA, Fahrenbruch CE, Olsufka M, et al. Changing incidence of out-of-hospital ventricular fibrillation, 1980–2000. JAMA 2002;288(23):3008–13.
3. Straus SM, Bleumink GS, Dieleman JP, et al. The incidence of sudden cardiac death in the general population. J Clin Epidemiol 2004;57(1):98–102.
4. Summaries for patients. Can stem cells restore cardiac tissue after a heart attack? Ann Intern Med 2004;140(9):I82.
5. Lloyd-Jones D, Adams RJ, Brown TM, et al. Executive summary: heart disease and stroke statistics—2010 update: a report from the American Heart Association. Circulation 2010;121(7):948–54.

6. Hypothermia after Cardiac Arrest Study Group. Mild therapeutic hypothermia to improve the neurologic outcome after cardiac arrest. N Engl J Med 2002;346(8): 549–56.

7. Bernard SA, Gray TW, Buist MD, et al. Treatment of comatose survivors of out-of-hospital cardiac arrest with induced hypothermia. N Engl J Med 2002; 346(8):557–63.

8. Field JM, Hazinski MF, Sayre MR, et al. Part 1: executive summary: 2010 American Heart Association Guidelines for Cardiopulmonary Resuscitation and Emergency Cardiovascular Care. Circulation 2010;122(18 Suppl 3):S640–56.

9. Oddo M, Ribordy V, Feihl F, et al. Early predictors of outcome in comatose survivors of ventricular fibrillation and non-ventricular fibrillation cardiac arrest treated with hypothermia: a prospective study. Crit Care Med 2008;36(8):2296–301.

10. Wolff B, Machill K, Schumacher D, et al. Early achievement of mild therapeutic hypothermia and the neurologic outcome after cardiac arrest. Int J Cardiol 2009; 133(2):223–8.

11. Gunn AJ. Cerebral hypothermia for prevention of brain injury following perinatal asphyxia. Curr Opin Pediatr 2000;12(2):111–5.

12. Hammer MD, Krieger DW. Hypothermia for acute ischemic stroke: not just another neuroprotectant. Neurologist 2003;9(6):280–9.

13. Sterz F, Zeiner A, Kurkciyan I, et al. Mild resuscitative hypothermia and outcome after cardiopulmonary resuscitation. J Neurosurg Anesthesiol 1996;8(1):88–96.

14. Nakashima K, Todd MM, Warner DS. The relation between cerebral metabolic rate and ischemic depolarization. A comparison of the effects of hypothermia, pentobarbital, and isoflurane. Anesthesiology 1995;82(5):1199–208.

15. Sakoh M, Gjedde A. Neuroprotection in hypothermia linked to redistribution of oxygen in brain. Am J Physiol Heart Circ Physiol 2003;285(1):H17–25.

16. Laptook AR, Corbett RJ, Burns D, et al. Neonatal ischemic neuroprotection by modest hypothermia is associated with attenuated brain acidosis. Stroke 1995; 26(7):1240–6.

17. Laptook AR, Corbett RJ, Sterett R, et al. Quantitative relationship between brain temperature and energy utilization rate measured in vivo using 31P and 1H magnetic resonance spectroscopy. Pediatr Res 1995;38(6):919–25.

18. Quinones-Hinojosa A, Malek JY, Ames A 3rd, et al. Metabolic effects of hypothermia and its neuroprotective effects on the recovery of metabolic and electrophysiological function in the ischemic retina in vitro. Neurosurgery 2003;52(5):1178–86 [discussion:1165–77].

19. Williams GD, Dardzinski BJ, Buckalew AR, et al. Modest hypothermia preserves cerebral energy metabolism during hypoxia-ischemia and correlates with brain damage: a 31P nuclear magnetic resonance study in unanesthetized neonatal rats. Pediatr Res 1997;42(5):700–8.

20. Gupta AK, Al-Rawi PG, Hutchinson PJ, et al. Effect of hypothermia on brain tissue oxygenation in patients with severe head injury. Br J Anaesth 2002;88(2):188–92.

21. Gunn AJ, Gunn TR. The 'pharmacology' of neuronal rescue with cerebral hypothermia. Early Hum Dev 1998;53(1):19–35.

22. Colbourne F, Sutherland G, Corbett D. Postischemic hypothermia. A critical appraisal with implications for clinical treatment. Mol Neurobiol 1997;14(3):171–201.

23. Small DL, Morley P, Buchan AM. Biology of ischemic cerebral cell death. Prog Cardiovasc Dis 1999;42(3):185–207.

24. Milde LN. Clinical use of mild hypothermia for brain protection: a dream revisited. J Neurosurg Anesthesiol 1992;4(3):211–5.

25. Polderman KH. Application of therapeutic hypothermia in the ICU: opportunities and pitfalls of a promising treatment modality. Part 1: indications and evidence. Intensive Care Med 2004;30(4):556–75.
26. Hagerdal M, Harp J, Nilsson L, et al. The effect of induced hypothermia upon oxygen consumption in the rat brain. J Neurochem 1975;24(2):311–6.
27. Palmer C, Vannucci RC, Christensen MA, et al. Regional cerebral blood flow and glucose utilization during hypothermia in newborn dogs. Anesthesiology 1989;71(5): 730–7.
28. Aoki M, Nomura F, Stromski ME, et al. Effects of pH on brain energetics after hypothermic circulatory arrest. Ann Thorac Surg 1993;55(5):1093–103.
29. Ehrlich MP, McCullough JN, Zhang N, et al. Effect of hypothermia on cerebral blood flow and metabolism in the pig. Ann Thorac Surg 2002;73(1):191–7.
30. Erecinska M, Thoresen M, Silver IA. Effects of hypothermia on energy metabolism in mammalian central nervous system. J Cereb Blood Flow Metab 2003;23(5):513–30.
31. Lanier WL. Cerebral metabolic rate and hypothermia: their relationship with ischemic neurologic injury. J Neurosurg Anesthesiol 1995;7(3):216–21.
32. Siesjo BK, Bengtsson F, Grampp W, et al. Calcium, excitotoxins, and neuronal death in the brain. Ann NY Acad Sci 1989;568:234–51.
33. Busto R, Globus MY, Dietrich WD, et al. Effect of mild hypothermia on ischemia-induced release of neurotransmitters and free fatty acids in rat brain. Stroke 1989; 20(7):904–10.
34. Illievich UM, Zornow MH, Choi KT, et al. Effects of hypothermic metabolic suppression on hippocampal glutamate concentrations after transient global cerebral ischemia. Anesth Analg 1994;78(5):905–11.
35. Komara JS, Nayini NR, Bialick HA, et al. Brain iron delocalization and lipid peroxidation following cardiac arrest. Ann Emerg Med 1986;15(4):384–9.
36. Bromont C, Marie C, Bralet J. Increased lipid peroxidation in vulnerable brain regions after transient forebrain ischemia in rats. Stroke 1989;20(7):918–24.
37. Katz LM, Young AS, Frank JE, et al. Regulated hypothermia reduces brain oxidative stress after hypoxic-ischemia. Brain Res 2004;1017(1-2):85–91.
38. Globus MY, Busto R, Lin B, et al. Detection of free radical activity during transient global ischemia and recirculation: effects of intraischemic brain temperature modulation. J Neurochem 1995;65(3):1250–6.
39. Globus MY, Alonso O, Dietrich WD, et al. Glutamate release and free radical production following brain injury: effects of posttraumatic hypothermia. J Neurochem 1995;65(4):1704–11.
40. Novack TA, Dillon MC, Jackson WT. Neurochemical mechanisms in brain injury and treatment: a review. J Clin Exp Neuropsychol 1996;18(5):685–706.
41. Raghupathi R, McIntosh TK. Pharmacotherapy for traumatic brain injury: a review. Proc West Pharmacol Soc 1998;41:241–6.
42. Xu L, Yenari MA, Steinberg GK, et al. Mild hypothermia reduces apoptosis of mouse neurons in vitro early in the cascade. J Cereb Blood Flow Metab 2002;22(1):21–8.
43. Povlishock JT, Buki A, Koiziumi H, et al. Initiating mechanisms involved in the pathobiology of traumatically induced axonal injury and interventions targeted at blunting their progression. Acta Neurochir Suppl 1999;73:15–20.
44. Adachi M, Sohma O, Tsuneishi S, et al. Combination effect of systemic hypothermia and caspase inhibitor administration against hypoxic-ischemic brain damage in neonatal rats. Pediatr Res 2001;50(5):590–5.
45. Raghupathi R, Graham DI, McIntosh TK. Apoptosis after traumatic brain injury. J Neurotrauma 2000;17(10):927–38.

46. Liou AK, Clark RS, Henshall DC, et al. To die or not to die for neurons in ischemia, traumatic brain injury and epilepsy: a review on the stress-activated signaling pathways and apoptotic pathways. Prog Neurobiol 2003;69(2):103–42.

47. Leker RR, Shohami E. Cerebral ischemia and trauma-different etiologies yet similar mechanisms: neuroprotective opportunities. Brain Res Brain Res Rev 2002;39(1): 55–73.

48. Callaway CW, Rittenberger JC, Logue ES, et al. Hypothermia after cardiac arrest does not alter serum inflammatory markers. Crit Care Med 2008;36(9):2607–12.

49. Schmidt OI, Heyde CE, Ertel W, et al. Closed head injury—an inflammatory disease? Brain Res Brain Res Rev 2005;48(2):388–99.

50. Merrill JE, Benveniste EN. Cytokines in inflammatory brain lesions: helpful and harmful. Trends Neurosci 1996;19(8):331–8.

51. Asensio VC, Campbell IL. Chemokines in the CNS: plurifunctional mediators in diverse states. Trends Neurosci 1999;22(11):504–12.

52. Wang GJ, Deng HY, Maier CM, et al. Mild hypothermia reduces ICAM-1 expression, neutrophil infiltration and microglia/monocyte accumulation following experimental stroke. Neuroscience 2002;114(4):1081–90.

53. Akriotis V, Biggar WD. The effects of hypothermia on neutrophil function in vitro. J Leukoc Biol 1985;37(1):51–61.

54. Dempsey RJ, Combs DJ, Maley ME, et al. Moderate hypothermia reduces postischemic edema development and leukotriene production. Neurosurgery 1987;21(2):177–81.

55. Fischer S, Clauss M, Wiesnet M, et al. Hypoxia induces permeability in brain microvessel endothelial cells via VEGF and NO. Am J Physiol 1999;276(4 Pt 1):C812–20.

56. Fischer S, Renz D, Wiesnet M, et al. Hypothermia abolishes hypoxia-induced hyperpermeability in brain microvessel endothelial cells. Brain Res Mol Brain Res 1999;74(1-2):135–44.

57. Huang ZG, Xue D, Preston E, et al. Biphasic opening of the blood–brain barrier following transient focal ischemia: effects of hypothermia. Can J Neurol Sci 1999; 26(4):298–304.

58. Chi OZ, Liu X, Weiss HR. Effects of mild hypothermia on blood-brain barrier disruption during isoflurane or pentobarbital anesthesia. Anesthesiology 2001;95(4): 933–8.

59. Smith SL, Hall ED. Mild pre- and posttraumatic hypothermia attenuates blood–brain barrier damage following controlled cortical impact injury in the rat. J Neurotrauma 1996;13(1):1–9.

60. Sterz F, Safar P, Tisherman S, et al. Mild hypothermic cardiopulmonary resuscitation improves outcome after prolonged cardiac arrest in dogs. Crit Care Med 1991;19(3): 379–89.

61. Markgraf CG, Clifton GL, Moody MR. Treatment window for hypothermia in brain injury. J Neurosurg 2001;95(6):979–83.

62. Nolan JP, Morley PT, Hoek TL, et al. Therapeutic hypothermia after cardiac arrest. An advisory statement by the Advancement Life support Task Force of the International Liaison committee on Resuscitation. Resuscitation 2003;57(3):231–5.

63. Silfvast T, Tiainen M, Poutiainen E, et al. Therapeutic hypothermia after prolonged cardiac arrest due to non-coronary causes. Resuscitation 2003;57(1):109–12.

64. Alzaga AG, Cerdan M, Varon J. Therapeutic hypothermia. Resuscitation 2006;70(3): 369–80.

65. Hossmann KA. Resuscitation potentials after prolonged global cerebral ischemia in cats. Crit Care Med 1988;16(10):964–71.

66. Danzl DF, Pozos RS. Accidental hypothermia. N Engl J Med 1994;331(26):1756–60.

67. Sterz F, Behringer W, Holzer M. Global hypothermia for neuroprotection after cardiac arrest. Acute Card Care 2006;8(1):25–30.
68. Nozari A, Safar P, Stezoski SW, et al. Critical time window for intra-arrest cooling with cold saline flush in a dog model of cardiopulmonary resuscitation. Circulation 2006;113(23):2690–6.
69. Polderman KH. Induced hypothermia and fever control for prevention and treatment of neurological injuries. Lancet 2008;371(9628):1955–69.
70. Polderman KH. Application of therapeutic hypothermia in the intensive care unit. Opportunities and pitfalls of a promising treatment modality—Part 2: practical aspects and side effects. Intensive Care Med 2004;30(5):757–69.
71. Polderman KH, Peerdeman SM, Girbes AR. Hypophosphatemia and hypomagnesemia induced by cooling in patients with severe head injury. J Neurosurg 2001;94(5):697–705.
72. Gal R, Slezak M, Zimova I, et al. Therapeutic hypothermia after out-of-hospital cardiac arrest with the target temperature 34–35 degrees C. Bratisl Lek Listy 2009;110(4):222–5.
73. Boddicker KA, Zhang Y, Zimmerman MB, et al. Hypothermia improves defibrillation success and resuscitation outcomes from ventricular fibrillation. Circulation 2005; 111(24):3195–201.
74. Dietrich WD, Busto R, Alonso O, et al. Intraischemic but not postischemic brain hypothermia protects chronically following global forebrain ischemia in rats. J Cereb Blood Flow Metab 1993;13(4):541–9.
75. Colbourne F, Corbett D. Delayed postischemic hypothermia: a six month survival study using behavioral and histological assessments of neuroprotection. J Neurosci 1995;15(11):7250–60.
76. Colbourne F, Corbett D. Delayed and prolonged post-ischemic hypothermia is neuroprotective in the gerbil. Brain Res 1994;654(2):265–72.
77. Hickey RW, Ferimer H, Alexander HL, et al. Delayed, spontaneous hypothermia reduces neuronal damage after asphyxial cardiac arrest in rats. Crit Care Med 2000;28(10):3511–6.
78. Shintani Y, Terao Y, Ohta H. Molecular mechanisms underlying hypothermia-induced neuroprotection. Stroke Res Treat 2010;2011:809–74.
79. Agnew DM, Koehler RC, Guerguerian AM, et al. Hypothermia for 24 hours after asphyxic cardiac arrest in piglets provides striatal neuroprotection that is sustained 10 days after rewarming. Pediatr Res 2003;54(2):253–62.
80. Markarian GZ, Lee JH, Stein DJ, et al. Mild hypothermia: therapeutic window after experimental cerebral ischemia. Neurosurgery 1996;38(3):542–50 [discussion: 551].
81. Polderman KH. Mechanisms of action, physiological effects, and complications of hypothermia. Crit Care Med 2009;37(7 Suppl):S186–202.
82. Busch M, Soreide E, Lossius HM, et al. Rapid implementation of therapeutic hypothermia in comatose out-of-hospital cardiac arrest survivors. Acta Anaesthesiol Scand 2006;50(10):1277–83.
83. Suehiro E, Povlishock JT. Exacerbation of traumatically induced axonal injury by rapid posthypothermic rewarming and attenuation of axonal change by cyclosporin A. J Neurosurg 2001;94(3):493–8.
84. Povlishock JT, Wei EP. Posthypothermic rewarming considerations following traumatic brain injury. J Neurotrauma 2009;26(3):333–40.
85. Leducq N, Delmas-Beauvieux MC, Bourdel-Marchasson I, et al. Mitochondrial permeability transition during hypothermic to normothermic reperfusion in rat liver demonstrated by the protective effect of cyclosporin A. Biochem J 1998;336(Pt 2):501–6.

86. Maxwell WL, Watson A, Queen R, et al. Slow, medium, or fast re-warming following post-traumatic hypothermia therapy? An ultrastructural perspective. J Neurotrauma 2005;22(8):873–84.

87. Alam HB, Rhee P, Honma K, et al. Does the rate of rewarming from profound hypothermic arrest influence the outcome in a swine model of lethal hemorrhage? J Trauma 2006;60(1):134–46.

88. Hildebrand F, van Griensven M, Giannoudis P, et al. Effects of hypothermia and re-warming on the inflammatory response in a murine multiple hit model of trauma. Cytokine 2005;31(5):382–93.

89. Kawahara F, Kadoi Y, Saito S, et al. Slow rewarming improves jugular venous oxygen saturation during rewarming. Acta Anaesthesiol Scand 2003;47(4):419–24.

90. Bissonnette B, Holtby HM, Davis AJ, et al. Cerebral hyperthermia in children after cardiopulmonary bypass. Anesthesiology 2000;93(3):611–8.

91. Janata A, Holzer M. Hypothermia after cardiac arrest. Prog Cardiovasc Dis 2009; 52(2):168–79.

92. Haugk M, Sterz F, Grassberger M, et al. Feasibility and efficacy of a new non-invasive surface cooling device in post-resuscitation intensive care medicine. Resuscitation 2007;75(1):76–81.

93. Proulx CI, Ducharme MB, Kenny GP. Safe cooling limits from exercise-induced hyperthermia. Eur J Appl Physiol 2006;96(4):434–45.

94. Schratter A, Weihs W, Holzer M, et al. External cardiac defibrillation during wet-surface cooling in pigs. Am J Emerg Med 2007;25(4):420–4.

95. Howes D, Ohley W, Dorian P, et al. Rapid induction of therapeutic hypothermia using convective-immersion surface cooling: safety, efficacy and outcomes. Resuscitation 2010;81(4):388–92.

96. Uray T, Malzer R. Out-of-hospital surface cooling to induce mild hypothermia in human cardiac arrest: a feasibility trial. Resuscitation 2008;77(3):331–8.

97. Tsai MS, Barbut D, Tang W, et al. Rapid head cooling initiated coincident with cardiopulmonary resuscitation improves success of defibrillation and post-resuscitation myocardial function in a porcine model of prolonged cardiac arrest. J Am Coll Cardiol 2008;51(20):1988–90.

98. Bernard S, Buist M, Monteiro O, et al. Induced hypothermia using large volume, ice-cold intravenous fluid in comatose survivors of out-of-hospital cardiac arrest: a preliminary report. Resuscitation 2003;56(1):9–13.

99. Kim F, Olsufka M, Carlbom D, et al. Pilot study of rapid infusion of 2 L of 4 degrees C normal saline for induction of mild hypothermia in hospitalized, comatose survivors of out-of-hospital cardiac arrest. Circulation 2005;112(5):715–9.

100. Kliegel A, Janata A, Wandaller C, et al. Cold infusions alone are effective for induction of therapeutic hypothermia but do not keep patients cool after cardiac arrest. Resuscitation 2007;73(1):46–53.

101. Kliegel A, Losert H, Sterz F, et al. Cold simple intravenous infusions preceding special endovascular cooling for faster induction of mild hypothermia after cardiac arrest—a feasibility study. Resuscitation 2005;64(3):347–51.

102. Polderman KH, Rijnsburger ER, Peerdeman SM, et al. Induction of hypothermia in patients with various types of neurologic injury with use of large volumes of ice-cold intravenous fluid. Crit Care Med 2005;33(12):2744–51.

103. Kim F, Olsufka M, Longstreth WT Jr, et al. Pilot randomized clinical trial of prehospital induction of mild hypothermia in out-of-hospital cardiac arrest patients with a rapid infusion of 4 degrees C normal saline. Circulation 2007;115(24):3064–70.

104. Bruel C, Parienti JJ, Marie W, et al. Mild hypothermia during advanced life support: a preliminary study in out-of-hospital cardiac arrest. Crit Care 2008;12(1):R31.

105. Kamarainen A, Virkkunen I, Tenhunen J, et al. Induction of therapeutic hypothermia during prehospital CPR using ice-cold intravenous fluid. Resuscitation 2008;79(2): 205–11.

106. Nordmark J, Rubertsson S. Induction of mild hypothermia with infusion of cold (4 degrees C) fluid during ongoing experimental CPR. Resuscitation 2005;66(3):357–65.

107. Riter HG, Brooks LA, Pretorius AM, et al. Intra-arrest hypothermia: both cold liquid ventilation with perfluorocarbons and cold intravenous saline rapidly achieve hypothermia, but only cold liquid ventilation improves resumption of spontaneous circulation. Resuscitation 2009;80(5):561–6.

108. Holzer M, Mullner M, Sterz F, et al. Efficacy and safety of endovascular cooling after cardiac arrest: cohort study and Bayesian approach. Stroke 2006;37(7):1792–7.

109. Al-Senani FM, Graffagnino C, Grotta JC, et al. A prospective, multicenter pilot study to evaluate the feasibility and safety of using the CoolGard System and Icy catheter following cardiac arrest. Resuscitation 2004;62(2):143–50.

110. Katz LM, Young A, Frank JE, et al. Neurotensin-induced hypothermia improves neurologic outcome after hypoxic-ischemia. Crit Care Med 2004;32(3):806–10.

111. Sun S, Tang W, Song F, et al. Pharmacologically induced hypothermia with cannabinoid receptor agonist WIN55, 212–2 after cardiopulmonary resuscitation. Crit Care Med 2010;38(12):2282–6.

112. Weng Y, Sun S, Song F, et al. Cholecystokinin octapeptide induces hypothermia and improves outcomes in a rat model of cardiopulmonary resuscitation. Crit Care Med 2011.

113. Holzer M, Behringer W, Janata A, et al. Extracorporeal venovenous cooling for induction of mild hypothermia in human-sized swine. Crit Care Med 2005;33(6): 1346–50.

114. Hong SB, Koh Y, Shim TS, et al. Physiologic characteristics of cold perfluorocarbon-induced hypothermia during partial liquid ventilation in normal rabbits. Anesth Analg 2002;94(1):157–62.

115. Staffey KS, Dendi R, Brooks LA, et al. Liquid ventilation with perfluorocarbons facilitates resumption of spontaneous circulation in a swine cardiac arrest model. Resuscitation 2008;78(1):77–84.

Protecting Mitochondrial Bioenergetic Function During Resuscitation from Cardiac Arrest

Raúl J. Gazmuri, MD, PhD, FCCM[a,b,]*, Jeejabai Radhakrishnan, PhD[a]

KEYWORDS
- Cardiopulmonary resuscitation • Energy metabolism
- Erythropoietin • Ischemia • Mitochondria • Myocardium
- Reperfusion injury • Sodium hydrogen antiporter
- Ventricular function

More than 90% of individuals who suffer an episode of out-of-hospital sudden cardiac arrest cannot be resuscitated by means of current cardiopulmonary resuscitation (CPR) techniques despite a large, sustained, coordinated, and costly public health effort that involves the community, emergency medical services, hospitals, and scientific institutions implementing evidence-based guidelines for resuscitation. The number of such victims is staggering, totaling more than 150,000 every year in the United States and many more worldwide.

Main barriers to improving survival after cardiac arrest include (1) the extremely narrow time window of only a few minutes available after cardiac arrest supervenes for deploying current resuscitation techniques before they become ineffective, (2) the limited hemodynamic capability of current resuscitation techniques to promote the levels of blood flow required to reverse ischemia of critical organs, and (3) the tissue injury—known as reperfusion injury—that stems from uncontrolled reintroduction of oxygen after ischemia. These are critical barriers that drive current resuscitation paradigms, forcing efforts to focus on minimizing delays in resuscitation at the scene

[a] Resuscitation Institute at Rosalind Franklin University of Medicine and Science, 3333 Green Bay Road, North Chicago, IL 60064, USA
[b] Medical Service, Captain James A. Lovell Federal Health Care Center, North Chicago, IL 60064, USA
* Corresponding author. Resuscitation Institute at Rosalind Franklin University of Medicine and Science, 3333 Green Bay Road, North Chicago, IL 60064.
E-mail address: raul.gazmuri@rosalindfranklin.edu

Crit Care Clin 28 (2012) 245–270
doi:10.1016/j.ccc.2012.02.001
0749-0704/12/$ – see front matter © 2012 Elsevier Inc. All rights reserved.

criticalcare.theclinics.com

and on devising approaches to augment the hemodynamic efficacy of the resuscitation efforts. Efforts to overcome the first two barriers coupled with improved post-resuscitation care—including hypothermia in unresponsive victims, percutaneous coronary interventions for suspected coronary etiology, and dedicated post-resuscitation critical care—have resulted in encouraging but modest increases in survival in recent years.

Growing basic and translational research supports that reperfusion injury can be attenuated through pharmacologic and nonpharmacologic interventions, resulting in improved resuscitation outcomes. Main contributors to reperfusion injury include Ca^{2+} overload[1,2] and generation of reactive oxygen species,[3] which exert injury mostly through compromising mitochondrial function. Recent studies aimed at examining the effects of protecting mitochondria from reperfusion injury during cardiac resuscitation indicate that preservation of mitochondrial bioenergetic function in the myocardium helps restoration of cardiac activity and sustained post-resuscitation circulation.

This article first provides a brief overview of mitochondria pertinent to their role in resuscitation followed by a discussion of myocardial abnormalities that occur during cardiac resuscitation and that could be minimized by interventions protecting mitochondrial bioenergetic function. These interventions represent work, mostly from our Resuscitation Institute, using inhibitors of the sodium–hydrogen exchanger isoform-1 (NHE-1) and erythropoietin.

MITOCHONDRIAL ANATOMY, FUNCTION, AND DYSFUNCTION

Consistent with their critical role in aerobic energy production, mitochondria are particularly abundant in tissues that have high metabolic activity. In the heart, approximately 35% of the cardiomyocyte volume is composed of mitochondria, which are "strategically" arranged in close proximity to the sarcomeres in a "crystal-like" structure with one mitochondrion per sarcomere[4] (**Fig. 1**A). Each mitochondrion has an outer and an inner membrane delimiting key functional components (**Fig. 1**B, C). The outer mitochondrial membrane is highly porous and provides the outer boundary of mitochondria. The inner mitochondrial membrane is highly tight and folds inwardly, forming convoluted loops known as cristae. These cristae enclose a space known as the intracristae space, which communicates with the intermembrane space through bottleneck-like junctions.[5,6] The space contained within the inner mitochondrial membrane is the matrix.

Energy Metabolism

The primary function of mitochondria is the generation of ATP through oxidative phosphorylation. The process starts with reduction of nicotinamide adenine dinucleotide (NAD^+) to NADH and flavin adenine dinucleotide (FAD) to $FADH_2$ during oxidation of pyruvate and citric acid cycle substrates. NADH and $FADH_2$ become oxidized again by transferring their electrons down a redox potential through complexes I, II, III, and IV of the electron transport chain (**Fig. 2**). The energy generated is used by complexes I, III, and IV—which are indeed proton pumps embedded in the inner mitochondrial membrane—to translocate H^+ from the matrix to outside the inner mitochondrial membrane against an electrochemical gradient, creating the proton motive force required for F_oF_1 ATPase to synthesize ATP from ADP and inorganic phosphate in the mitochondrial matrix. The newly synthesized ATP is then exchanged for ADP through the inner mitochondrial membrane by the adenine nucleotide translocator (ANT) and is used to phosphorylate creatine into phosphocreatine, which is then exported outside the mitochondria to power energy-requiring processes.

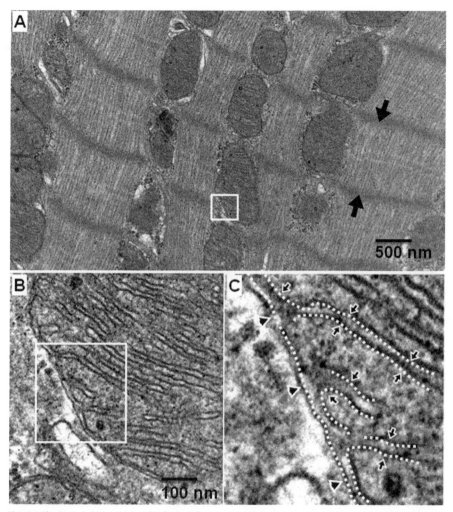

Fig. 1. Electron micrograph of left ventricular mitochondria isolated from a Sprague-Dawley retired breeder rat at the Resuscitation Institute. (*A*) Intermyofibrillar mitochondria orderly organized within the zone demarcated by two Z lines (*black arrowheads*), the structure where adjacent sarcomeres connect and thin filaments anchor. (*B, C*) Higher magnification of section in mitochondrion selected in (*A*) showing the outer mitochondrial membrane (*arrowheads*) and the inner mitochondrial membrane folding inside the mitochondrial matrix.

Oxygen plays an essential role in energy generation as the final acceptor of electrons from the electron transport chain. Interruption in oxygen delivery (eg, after onset of cardiac arrest) halts electron flow, precluding generation of the proton motive force required for ATP synthesis. Cells can still generate ATP "anaerobically" but at a much lower rate that is not sufficient to meet metabolic demands. ATP is generated anaerobically through glycolysis, with lactate as the final product, which diffuses outside the cell and can be readily measured and used as a marker of ischemia and its reversal. ATP can also be regenerated anaerobically from cellular stores of phosphocreatine, but this is a nonregenerative mechanism and is rapidly exhausted.

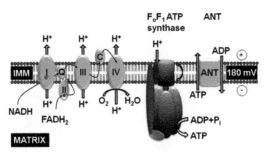

Fig. 2. Schematic rendition of key mitochondrial components involved in ATP synthesis via oxidative phosphorylation. ANT, adenine nucleotide translocator; C, cytochrome c; e, electrons; IMM, inner mitochondrial membrane; I, II, III, and IV, respiratory chain complexes; Q, coenzyme Q.

Accordingly, after cardiac arrest, an intense energy deficit develops in metabolically active organs—heart and brain—that precludes maintaining their function. Cardiopulmonary resuscitation becomes the means to reoxygenate and restore mitochondrial bioenergetic function. However, as previously stated, reoxygenation is accompanied by reperfusion injury that, in turn, may compromise mitochondrial bioenergetic function. Much of the work discussed in this article provides evidence supporting the concept that resuscitation can be facilitated by protecting mitochondrial bioenergetic function.

Cytochrome c Release as a Marker of Mitochondrial Injury

This brief synopsis of mitochondrial function, however, would not be complete if the role of mitochondria in modulating cell viability and eventual cell death is not addressed. It is now well established that mitochondria can signal cell death through the release of various pro-apoptotic proteins, including cytochrome c, apoptosis-inducing factor, Smac/DIABLO, endonuclease G, and a serine protease Omi/HtrA2.[7,8] Of these proteins, cytochrome c has been the most widely investigated.

Cytochrome c is a 14-kDa hemoprotein normally present in the intracristae space and the intermembrane space attached to the inner mitochondrial membrane loosely bound to cardiolipin (see **Fig. 2**). Cytochrome c plays a key physiologic role enabling electron transfer from complex III to complex IV. However, cytochrome c, through various pathologic mechanisms, can be released to the cytosol including ultraviolet irradiation,[9] serum deprivation,[10] growth factor withdrawal,[10–12] and also conditions present during ischemia and reperfusion such as Ca^{2+} overload,[13] hypoxia,[14] and generation of reactive oxygen species.[15]

In our laboratory, we reported using a rat model of ventricular fibrillation (VF) that cytochrome c is released to the cytosol after resuscitation from cardiac arrest, where it activates the "intrinsic" or "mitochondrial" apoptotic pathway through formation of an oligomeric complex known as the apoptosome.[16] The apoptosome activates caspase-9 which, in turn, activates downstream executioner caspases 3, 6, and 7.[17] Activation of these executioner caspases can lead to apoptotic cell death.[18] However, in our rat model activation of the mitochondrial apoptotic pathway did not cause cell death or was responsible for the severe myocardial dysfunction that occurs post-resuscitation, at least within the initial 4 hours after return of spontaneous circulation.[19,20]

Cytochrome c can also "leak" into the bloodstream under conditions associated with mitochondrial injury such as chemotherapy,[21,22] acute myocardial infarction,[23]

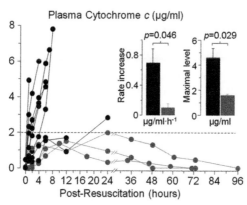

Fig. 3. Serial measurements of plasma cytochrome *c* by reverse-phase HPLC in rats successfully resuscitated after 8 minutes of untreated ventricular fibrillation. Measurements were made until cytochrome *c* levels had returned to baseline or the rat had died. Gray symbols represent survivors (n = 3); black symbols represent nonsurvivors (n = 9). (*From* Ayoub IM, Radhakrishnan J, Gazmuri RJ. Targeting mitochondria for resuscitation from cardiac arrest. Crit Care Med 2008;36:S440–6; with permission.)

the systemic inflammatory response syndrome,[24] and influenza-associated encephalopathy.[25,26] Studies in our laboratory further demonstrate that cytochrome *c* can be also released to the bloodstream after resuscitation from cardiac arrest.[19] In these studies, plasma cytochrome *c* was serially measured using reverse-phase high-performance liquid chromatography (HPLC) in rats successfully resuscitated from VF. In survivors, plasma cytochrome *c* gradually increased to levels that did not exceed 2 μg/mL, returning to baseline within 48 to 96 hours. In nonsurvivors, cytochrome *c* increased at a faster rate and attained levels that substantially exceeded those observed in survivors without reversal before demise from cardiovascular dysfunction (**Fig. 3**). These observations support the idea that plasma cytochrome *c* could be a marker of mitochondrial injury and used to assess the effect of interventions designed to protect mitochondria during cardiac resuscitation.

Two main mechanisms have been proposed to explain cytochrome *c* release from mitochondria; namely, opening of the mitochondrial permeability transition pore (mPTP) and selective permeabilization of the outer mitochondrial membrane. mPTP opening is typically triggered by abnormalities central to ischemia and reperfusion injury including Ca^{2+} overload, production of reactive oxygen species, depletion of ATP and ADP, and increases in inorganic phosphate.[27] mPTP opening allows molecules up to 1500 Da to enter the mitochondrial matrix along with water and solutes, causing mitochondrial swelling, unfolding of the inner mitochondrial membrane cristae, and disruption of the outer mitochondrial membrane, ultimately precipitating cytochrome *c* release to the cytosol.[27,28] mPTP opening also causes collapse of the electrochemical gradient across the inner mitochondrial membrane, uncoupling oxidative phosphorylation. In addition, release of cytochrome *c* could also occur through selective permeabilization of the outer mitochondrial membrane associated with oligomerization and formation of channel-like structures by proteins of the B-cell lymphoma-2 (Bcl-2) family.[29,30] Release of cytochrome *c* is further facilitated during ischemia and reperfusion by peroxidation of cardiolipin consequent to mitochondrial Ca^{2+} overload and production of reactive oxygen species.[31–33]

Cardiolipin is the principal lipid constituent of the inner mitochondrial membrane, and to which a fraction of cytochrome *c* is bound.

MYOCARDIAL ABNORMALITIES DURING CARDIAC RESUSCITATION

The working heart is a highly metabolic organ that under normal resting conditions extracts nearly 70% of the oxygen supplied by the coronary circulation[34,35] representing close to 10% of the total body oxygen consumption. However, the heart has minimal capability for extracting additional oxygen such that increases in metabolic demands can be met only by autoregulatory increases in coronary blood flow through vasodilation of the coronary circuit.[36] Consequently, a severe energy imbalance develops when cardiac arrest occurs and coronary blood flow ceases. The severe energy imbalance continues during the ensuing resuscitation effort when current closed-chest resuscitation techniques are used because of the very limited capability for generating systemic and coronary blood flow.[37]

The magnitude of the energy imbalance is contingent on the metabolic requirements and is particularly severe in the presence of VF when the oxygen requirements are comparable to or exceed those of the beating heart.[38,39] A lesser energy deficit is expected during cardiac arrest with a quiescent or minimally active heart (ie, asystole or pulseless electrical activity precipitated by asphyxia or exsanguination).

Various functional myocardial abnormalities develop during cardiac arrest and resuscitation that are detrimental to cardiac resuscitation. These abnormalities include reductions in left ventricular distensibility during the resuscitation effort followed by reperfusion arrhythmias and post-resuscitation myocardial dysfunction.

Left Ventricular Distensibility

Studies in various animal models of VF and resuscitation have shown progressive thickening of the left ventricular wall accompanied by parallel reductions in left ventricular cavity without changes in intracavitary pressures during cardiac resuscitation.[40,41] A functionally similar phenomenon known as ischemic contracture was reported in the early 1970s during open heart surgery when operations were conducted under normothermic conditions in fibrillating hearts[42,43] and more recently after prolonged intervals of untreated VF.[44] However, ischemic contracture is associated with profound reductions in myocardial ATP and often leads to a "stony heart" heralding irreversible ischemic injury.[45] Reductions in left ventricular distensibility observed during cardiac resuscitation is a different phenomenon: (1) it occurs much earlier than the "stony heart" starting coincident with reperfusion during the resuscitation effort;[40,41] (2) it is associated with less ATP depletion;[46] (3) it has been attributed to myocardial energy deficit compounded by cytosolic and mitochondrial Ca^{2+} overload precluding complete relaxation of individual cardiomyocytes; (4) it evolves into diastolic dysfunction upon return of spontaneous circulation;[47] (5) it is largely reversible;[48] and (6) it is amenable to therapeutic intervention (**Fig. 4**).

Reductions in left ventricular distensibility adversely affect the ability of chest compression to generate forward blood flow. As blood returns to the heart during the relaxation phase of chest compression, distensible ventricles are important to properly accommodate the returning blood and establish an adequate preload for the subsequent compression. Progressive reductions in left ventricular distensibility during chest compression contribute to progressive reduction in the hemodynamic efficacy of closed-chest resuscitation. Studies in a porcine model of VF have shown that the severity of this phenomenon is proportional to the duration of untreated VF.[40]

Work in our laboratory demonstrates that reductions in left ventricular distensibility can be prevented by pharmacologic interventions targeting reperfusion injury leading

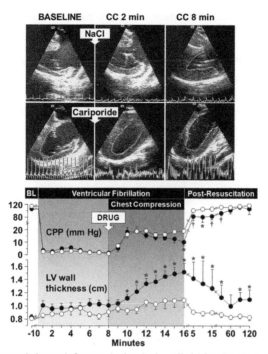

Fig. 4. The upper panel shows left ventricular (LV) wall thickening in a control pig (*upper frames*) but not in a pig treated with cariporide (lower frames). The images were obtained by transesophageal echocardiography at the end of mechanical diastole (baseline, BL) and at the end of "compression diastole" at 2 and 8 minutes of chest compression (CC). The endocardial border was delineated to facilitate visualization. The lower panel shows progressive decreases in the coronary perfusion pressure (CPP) coincident with progressive thickening of the left ventricular wall in pigs that received 0.9 % NaCl (*closed symbols*, n = 8) but not in pigs that received cariporide (*open symbols*, n = 8). NaCl or cariporide (drug, 3 mg/kg) was given immediately before starting chest compression. Values are mean ± SEM. *P<.05, †P<.001 vs cariporide by one-way ANOVA. (*From* Ayoub IM, Kolarova JD, Yi Z, et al. Sodium-hydrogen exchange inhibition during ventricular fibrillation: beneficial effects on ischemic contracture, action potential duration, reperfusion arrhythmias, myocardial function, and resuscitability. Circulation 2003;107:1804–9; with permission.)

to hemodynamically more stable closed-chest resuscitation as discuss in the subsequent sections.[41,49]

In humans, Takino and Okada[50] reported on 59 adult patients who suffered nontraumatic out-of-hospital cardiac arrest and underwent open-chest direct manual cardiac compression in the emergency department after failure of closed-chest resuscitation. A "firm" myocardium was noticed during manual cardiac compression in 36 cases affecting predominantly the left ventricle. In the remaining 23 cases the hearts were "soft." Takino and Okada also noted that some hearts became "firm" during compression.

The presence of a "firm" myocardium was associated with reduced hemodynamic efficacy of cardiac compression as evidenced by a lower end-tidal CO_2 tension ($P_{ET}CO_2$), which is a well-documented surrogate measurement of systemic and regional blood flow during cardiac resuscitation.[37,51–53] Hearts with "very firm" myocardium never regained spontaneous contractions. Hearts with "less firm" myocardium showed some, albeit insufficient, spontaneous contractions. Hearts with "soft" myocardium regained contractions and were able to generate a peripheral pulse in most instances.

Reperfusion Arrhythmias

Premature ventricular complexes and episodes of ventricular tachycardia and VF commonly occur during the early minutes after return of cardiac activity. Post-resuscitation episodes of VF—which require additional electrical shocks—have been reported in up to 79% of patients, with some studies showing an inverse relationship between the number of episodes and survival.[54] The underlying cell mechanisms are complex but prominently involve cytosolic Ca^{2+} overload and afterdepolarizations. There are repolarization abnormalities that include shortening of the action potential duration, decreased action potential amplitude, and development of action potential alternans creating conditions for reentry. Experimentally, these repolarization abnormalities are short lived (5–10 minutes) and coincide with the interval of increased propensity for ventricular arrhythmias and recurrent VF.[41] These repolarization abnormalities and reperfusion arrhythmias can be markedly attenuated by NHE-1 inhibition.[41]

Post-Resuscitation Myocardial Dysfunction

Variable degrees of systolic[55–58] and diastolic[41,59] dysfunction develop after resuscitation from cardiac arrest. Dysfunction occurs despite full restoration of coronary blood flow and is largely reversible, conforming to the definition of myocardial stunning. Systolic dysfunction is characterized by decreases in contractility—documented by load-independent indices derived from varying end-systolic pressure–volume relationship—leading to reductions left ventricular ejection fraction, cardiac index, left ventricular stroke work,[56,57] and poor tolerance to afterload increases.[60] Diastolic dysfunction is characterized by left ventricular wall thickening with reductions in end-diastolic volume and impaired relaxation.[41] Diastolic dysfunction appears to be maximal immediately after restoration of spontaneous circulation, with the magnitude of wall thickness correlating closely with wall thickness during VF,[47] suggesting a common pathogenic thread. From a functional perspective, diastolic dysfunction may limit the compensatory ventricular dilatation required to overcome decreases in contractility according to the Frank–Starling mechanism.

Myocardial dysfunction is characteristically responsive to inotropic stimulation and therefore pump function can be improved by administration of agents such as β-agonists (ie, dobutamine) and phosphodiesterase inhibitors (ie, milrinone). Dobutamine acts primarily on β_1, β_2, and α_1 receptors. Its hemodynamic effects include increases in stroke volume and cardiac output with decreases in systemic and pulmonary vascular resistance. Studies in animal models of cardiac arrest have demonstrated substantial reversal of post-resuscitation systolic and diastolic dysfunction using doses ranging from 5 to 10 $\mu g/kg \cdot min^{-1}$.[61–63] However, a dose of 5 $\mu g/kg \cdot min^{-1}$ was found in domestic pigs (24 ± 0.4 kg) to provide the best balance by restoring post-resuscitation systolic and diastolic function without adverse effects on myocardial oxygen consumption.[62] Phosphodiesterase inhibitors such as milrinone also exert inotropic and vasodilator effects and have been shown experimentally to improve post-resuscitation myocardial dysfunction.[64] However, the effectiveness of conventional the inotropic agents may be limited by effects on heart rate and the possibility of worsening ischemic injury in settings of critically reduced coronary artery blood flow.

INTERVENTIONS TARGETING MITOCHONDRIAL FUNCTION

Two lines of research at the Resuscitation Institute support the feasibility of targeting mitochondrial bioenergetic function for resuscitation from cardiac arrest. One line relates to work using NHE-1 inhibitors in various animal models of cardiac arrest over a period of approximately 10 years.[41,46,49,65–70] The other line relates to more recent work using erythropoietin in a rat model of cardiac arrest[71] and in a small clinical study in patients suffering out-of-hospital cardiac arrest.[72] Both lines of research support the rationale and feasibility of using either an NHE-1 inhibitor or erythropoietin for preservation of left ventricular myocardial distensibility during cardiac resuscitation.

NHE-1 Inhibitors

Mechanisms of injury

The intense myocardial ischemia that develops shortly after the onset of cardiac arrest prompts profound and sustained intracellular acidosis.[73–75] Intracellular acidosis activates the sarcolemmal NHE-1, initiating an electroneutral $Na^+–H^+$ exchange that brings Na^+ into the cell.[76] During the ensuing resuscitation effort, the myocardium is reperfused with blood that typically has a normal pH resulting in the washout of protons accumulated in the extracellular space during the preceding interval of ischemia, intensifying the sarcolemmal $Na^+–H^+$ exchange and the resulting Na^+ entry.[65,76,77] Na^+ accumulates in the cytosol because the Na^+,K^+-ATPase activity is concomitantly reduced,[78] such that progressive and prominent increases in cytosolic Na^+ occurs. Na^+ may also enter the cell through Na^+ channels and the $Na^+–HCO_3^-$ cotransporter. The cytosolic Na^+ excess, in turn, drives sarcolemmal Ca^{2+} influx through reverse mode operation of the sarcolemmal $Na^+–Ca^{2+}$ exchanger, leading to cytosolic and mitochondrial Ca^{2+} overload,[79] causing a myriad of detrimental effects.

Ca^{2+} entering mitochondria can be sequestered in large amounts through a process that involves influx through the Ca^{2+} uniporter and efflux through the $Na^+–Ca^{2+}$ exchanger.[80] However, as mitochondrial Ca^{2+} rises the mitochondrial $Na^+–Ca^{2+}$ exchanger becomes saturated and mitochondrial Ca^{2+} overload occurs.[80] Mitochondrial Ca^{2+} overload can compromise the capability of mitochondria to sustain oxidative phosphorylation[81] and also promote the release of pro-apoptotic factors including cytochrome c.[82]

The relevance of this mechanism of injury is highlighted by a large series of preclinical studies demonstrating consistent attenuation of myocardial injury caused by ischemia and reperfusion when sarcolemmal Na^+ entry is limited.[76,83,84]

Effects of NHE–1 inhibitors on resuscitation

Research using various rat and pig models of cardiac arrest support a consistent myocardial benefit associated with inhibition of NHE-1 activity during resuscitation from VF, including preservation of left ventricular distensibility, attenuation of reperfusion arrhythmias, and amelioration of post-resuscitation myocardial dysfunction, all favoring improved resuscitability and survival.[41,46,49,65–70,85–87]

Effects on left ventricular distensibility

The initial findings suggesting that NHE-1 inhibition could attenuate reductions in left ventricular distensibility during resuscitation and also prevent post-resuscitation diastolic dysfunction were made using an isolated (Langendorff) rat model of VF and simulated resuscitation.[65,66] As shown in **Fig. 5**, infusion of the NHE-1 inhibitor cariporide during simulated resuscitation markedly attenuated left ventricular pressure increases, consistent with preservation of left ventricular distensibility. Post-resuscitation,

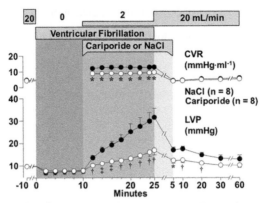

Fig. 5. Isolated perfused rat heart model of VF and simulated resuscitation. Upper horizontal bars represent perfusate flow, VF, and duration of cariporide or NaCl infusion. CVR denotes coronary vascular resistance; LVP, left ventricular end-diastolic pressure during sinus rhythm and "arrest" pressure during VF. Values are mean ± SEM. Closed symbols denote NaCl and open symbols cariporide. Differences in LVP and CVR between treatment groups were significant ($P<.0001$ by two-way ANOVA for treatment effect). *$P<.05$, †$P<.01$, ‡$P<.001$ vs NaCl by one-way ANOVA. (*Adapted from* Gazmuri RJ, Ayoub IM, Hoffner E, et al. Successful ventricular defibrillation by the selective sodium-hydrogen exchanger isoform-1 inhibitor cariporide. Circulation 2001;104:234–9; with permission.)

the end-diastolic left ventricle pressure–volume relationship was preserved at baseline levels (**Fig. 6**). Cariporide elicited the effects despite administration starting after 10 minutes of untreated VF, supporting the clinical relevance of the findings.

Subsequent studies in a pig model of VF and closed-chest resuscitation paralleled the findings in the isolated rat heart showing preservation of left ventricular wall thickness and cavity size (see **Fig. 4**; data on cavity size not shown).[41] Preservation of left ventricular myocardial distensibility enabled the

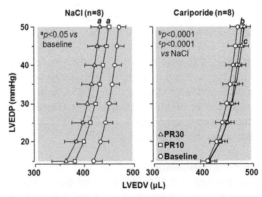

Fig. 6. Left ventricular end-diastolic pressure (LVEDP)–volume (LVEDV) curves. PR denotes post-resuscitation at 10 and 30 minutes. Measurements made in hearts from **Fig. 3**. (*Adapted from* Gazmuri RJ, Ayoub IM, Hoffner E, et al. Successful ventricular defibrillation by the selective sodium-hydrogen exchanger isoform-1 inhibitor cariporide. Circulation 2001;104: 234–9; with permission.)

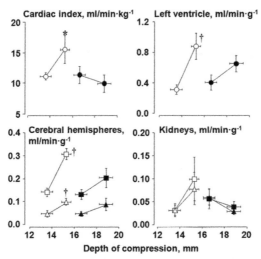

Fig. 7. Cardiac index and organ blood flow as a function of depth of compression in rats during VF and closed-chest resuscitation. Rats were randomized to receive a bolus of cariporide (*open symbols*) or vehicle control (*closed symbols*) at the start of chest compression. The first symbol represents data from series 1 and the second symbol data from series 2. For paired organs, triangles denote right and squares left. Values are mean ± SEM. *$P<.05$ vs 0.9% NaCl by one-way ANOVA in series 2; †$P<.01$ vs series 1 within each treatment group by one-way ANOVA. (*Adapted from* Kolarova JD, Ayoub IM, Gazmuri RJ. Cariporide enables hemodynamically more effective chest compression by leftward shift of its flow-depth relationship. Am J Physiol Heart Circ Physiol 2005;288:H2904–11; with permission.)

generation of higher coronary perfusion pressures (CPPs), prompting higher resuscitability rates (2/8 vs 8/8; $P<.05$).[41]

We then reasoned that if left ventricular myocardial distensibility—and therefore preload—could be preserved by NHE-1 inhibition then higher forward blood flows could be generated for a given compression depth, thus enhancing the relationship between forward blood flow and compression depth.

Studies were performed measuring systemic and organ blood flow using fluorescent microspheres in an rat model of VF and closed-chest resuscitation.[49] Two series of 14 experiments each were conducted in which rats were subjected to 10 minutes of untreated VF followed by 8 minutes of chest compression before defibrillation was attempted. Compression depth was adjusted to maintain an aortic diastolic pressure between 26 and 28 mm Hg in the first series and between 36 and 38 mm Hg in the second series. Within each series, rats were randomized to receive cariporide (3 mg/kg) or NaCl 0.9% (control) before chest compression was started. In rats that received cariporide, the compression depth required to generate a given systemic and organ blood flow was markedly reduced compared with that in rats that received the vehicle control (**Fig. 7**). Thus, a higher forward blood flow leading to higher regional organ blood flows could be generated for a given depth of compression in the presence of cariporide.

We further reasoned that administration of a vasopressor agent in the presence of an NHE-1 inhibitor could result in a higher systemic and CPP for the simple reason that pressure is a function of flow and resistance. This was indeed the case, as demonstrated in a rat model of VF and closed-chest resuscitation.[68] The studies

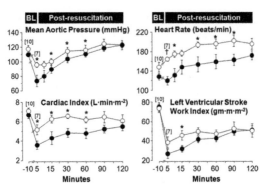

Fig. 8. Baseline and post-resuscitation left ventricular and hemodynamic function in pigs randomized to receive cariporide (*open symbols*) or 0.9% NaCl (*closed symbols*). Numbers in brackets indicate sample size. Values are mean ± SEM. *$P<.05$; †$P<.001$ vs 0.9% NaCl analyzed by one-way ANOVA. (*Adapted from* Ayoub IM, Kolarova J, Gazmuri RJ. Cariporide given during resuscitation promotes return of electrically stable and mechanically competent cardiac activity. Resuscitation 2009;81:106–10; with permission.)

involved two series of 16 experiments each using epinephrine in one series and vasopressin in the other. Within each series rats were randomized to receive cariporide or NaCl control. A significantly higher CPP was elicited with either vasopressor agent in rats that had received cariporide. A similar effect was observed associated with the administration of epinephrine in a pig model of VF and closed-chest resuscitation.[69] These effects on CPP are important; if translated clinically they could be highly relevant because only small increases in CPP are required to have a dramatic effect on resuscitability.[88]

Effects on post-resuscitation arrhythmias and refibrillation
NHE-1 inhibition using cariporide was markedly effective in suppressing ventricular ectopic activity during the early post-resuscitation period.[41,66,69,86] This effect was associated with preservation of the action potential duration,[42] an effect that could reduce the risk of reentry minimizing the risk of VF during the early post-resuscitation interval.[86] This is an important effect, which if translated clinically could help stabilize initially resuscitated victim of out-of-hospital cardiac arrest and avert recurrent episodes of cardiac arrest during initial post-resuscitation period while en route to a hospital.

Effects on post-resuscitation myocardial function
Several series in rat and pig models of VF and resuscitation have shown beneficial effects of NHE-1 inhibitors on post-resuscitation myocardial function (**Fig. 8**) using cariporide in a pig model of VF and closed-chest resuscitation.[86] A similar post-resuscitation benefit was observed using the NHE-1 inhibitor zoniporide in an open-chest pig model of resuscitation by extracorporeal circulation.[46] This effect translated to improved short-term survival in a rat model of VF and closed-chest resuscitation.[87]

Mechanisms of the resuscitation effects
Effects on cytosolic Na⁺ and mitochondrial Ca²⁺. A rat model of VF and closed-chest resuscitation was used to examine the effects of NHE-1 inhibition and of Na⁺ channel

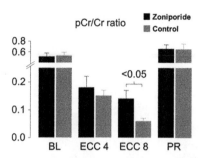

Fig. 9. Myocardial measurements in pigs randomly assigned to receive 3 mg/kg of zoniporide (*black bars*) or 0.9% NaCl (*gray bars*) after 8 minutes of untreated VF before start of extracorporeal circulation (ECC). Measurements were obtained at baseline (BL), during VF at ECC 4 and 8 minutes, and at 60 minutes post-resuscitation (PR). Each group had eight pigs at baseline and ECC and six pigs in the zoniporide group and five in the NaCl group at PR. Values are mean ± SEM. (*Adapted from* Ayoub IM, Kolarova J, Kantola R, et al. Zoniporide preserves left ventricular compliance during ventricular fibrillation and minimizes post-resuscitation myocardial dysfunction through benefits on energy metabolism. Crit Care Med 2007;35: 2329–36; with permission.)

blockade (interventions collectively referred to as "Na$^+$-limiting interventions") on intracellular Na$^+$, mitochondrial Ca^{2+}, cardiac function, and plasma levels of cardio-specific troponin I (cTnI) after resuscitation.[70] Limiting sarcolemmal Na$^+$ entry attenuated increases in cytosolic Na$^+$ and mitochondrial Ca^{2+}overload during chest compression and the post-resuscitation phase. Attenuation of cytosolic Na$^+$ and mitochondrial Ca^{2+} increases was accompanied by preservation of left ventricular myocardial distensibility during chest compression, less post-resuscitation myocardial dysfunction, and lower levels of cardiospecific troponin I.

Effects on energy metabolism. An open-chest pig model of electrically induced VF and extracorporeal circulation was developed to study the myocardial energy effects of inhibiting NHE-1 under conditions of controlled CPP.[46] VF was induced by epicardial delivery of an alternating current and left untreated for 8 minutes. Extra-corporeal circulation was then started with the flow adjusted to maintain a CPP at 10 mm Hg for 10 minutes before defibrillation and restoration of spontaneous circulation were attempted. The target CPP was chosen to mimic the low CPP generated by closed-chest resuscitation. Two groups of eight pigs each were randomized to receive the NHE-1 inhibitor zoniporide (3 mg/kg) or vehicle control as a right atrial bolus immediately before extracorporeal circulation was started. Like in a previous study using the NHE-1 inhibitor cariporide[41] (see **Fig. 4**), zoniporide also prevented progressive reductions in cavity size and progressive thickening of the left ventricular wall.

The myocardial effects occurred without changes in coronary blood flow or coronary vascular resistance, indicating that the favorable myocardial effects of NHE-1 inhibition during resuscitation were not likely the result of increased blood flow and oxygen availability (eg, by less extrinsic compression of the coronary circuit).

Myocardial tissue measurements indicated that administration of zoniporide prevented progressive loss of oxidative phosphorylation during the interval of simulated resuscitation. Animals that received zoniporide (1) maintained a higher creatine phosphate-to-creatine (pCr/Cr) ratio as shown in **Fig. 9**, (2) maintained a higher

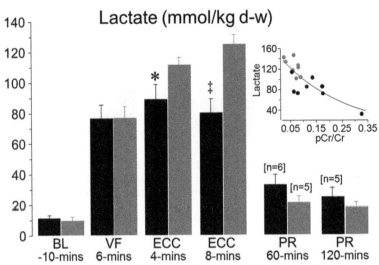

Fig. 10. Myocardial lactate measurements in experiments described in **Fig. 9**. Numbers in brackets indicate when sample size decreased from the initial 8 or preceding ones. Insert shows the relationship between lactate and pCr/Cr ratio at ECC 8 minutes. The regression line represents an exponential decay function ($R^2 = 0.63$, $P<.001$). Values are mean $\pm$ SEM. *$P<.05$, ‡$P<.001$ vs NaCl by Student t-test. (*Adapted from* Ayoub IM, Kolarova J, Kantola R, et al. Zoniporide preserves left ventricular compliance during ventricular fibrillation and minimizes post-resuscitation myocardial dysfunction through benefits on energy metabolism. Crit Care Med 2007;35:2329–36; with permission.)

ATP/ADP ratio, and (3) had lesser increases in adenosine. These measurements are consistent with regeneration of ADP into ATP by mitochondria instead of downstream degradation into adenosine, with the newly formed ATP being used to regenerate creatinine phosphate, all indicative of preserved mitochondrial bioenergetic function. These changes were accompanied by prominent amelioration of myocardial lactate increases, attaining levels that were inversely proportional to the pCr/Cr ratio at 8 minutes of VF and ECC, suggesting a shift away from anaerobic metabolism consequent to preservation of mitochondrial bioenergetic function in pigs treated with zoniporide (**Fig. 10**).

These energy effects are consistent with NHE-1 inhibition protecting mitochondrial bioenergetic function—probably as a result of limiting mitochondrial Ca^{2+} overload—and supportive of the concept that left ventricular myocardial distensibility during resuscitation is likely to be preserved by activating mitochondrial mechanisms capable of maintaining bioenergetic function.

Erythropoietin

Because development of NHE-1 inhibitors for clinical use has been driven by indications other than resuscitation, and these efforts have been unsuccessful so far, we sought alternative, clinically available, compounds that could elicit similar mitochondrial effect within a time window relevant to resuscitation. One of these compounds is erythropoietin.

Erythropoietin is a 30.4-kDa glycoprotein best known for its action on erythroid progenitor cells and regulation of circulating red cell mass. However, several studies have recently shown that erythropoietin also activates potent cell survival mechanisms during ischemia and reperfusion through genomic and nongenomic signaling mechanisms in a broad array of organs and tissues including the heart,[89-98] brain,[99-102] spinal cord,[103] kidney,[104,105] liver,[105] and skin.[106]

The action of erythropoietin begins with binding to a specific cell membrane receptor known as the erythropoietin receptor (EpoR). This receptor is a member of the type I superfamily of single-transmembrane cytokine receptors. Erythropoietin binding to EpoR triggers cross-phosphorylation and activation of Janus tyrosine kinases (JAK) 1 and 2. JAK activation, in turn, prompts phosphorylation of tyrosine residues present in the EpoR intracellular domains, creating docking sites for the recruitment and activation of multiple signaling proteins that have Src-homology-2 (SH2) domains resulting in well-known anti-apoptotic,[92] anti-inflammatory,[107,108] and proliferative effects.[109,110] The time course of these effects vary contingent on the specific signaling mechanism and the duration of the erythropoietin–EpoR binding.

Without negating the potential benefits of the anti-apoptotic, anti-inflammatory, and proliferative effects of erythropoietin effects, we have been interested in mechanisms responsible for "rapid" activation of cell protective mechanisms. Erythropoietin activates signaling pathways that converge on mitochondria and that favor preservation of bioenergetic function in spite of the adverse conditions present during ischemia and reperfusion. These signaling pathways are likely to involve activation of protein kinase C epsilon (PKCε) and protein kinase B (Akt) with translocation from the cytosol to mitochondria.

PKCε activation is a well-established mechanism of myocardial protection linked to preconditioning and acute protection.[111] PKCε is located primarily in the cytosol and it is activated by phosphorylation through various signaling mechanisms, including erythropoietin. Erythropoietin mediates the effect through phosphorylation of phosphoinositide-dependent kinase-1 (PDK$_1$) on activation of phosphatidyl inositide kinase (PI3K), which is an SH2 domain containing signaling protein. Phosphorylated PKCε translocates to the mitochondria, where it signals opening of putative mitochondrial ATP-sensitive K$^+$ channels (K$_{ATP}$ channels),[112,113] activation of the mitochondrial enzymes cytochrome c oxidase[114] and aldehyde dehydrogease,[115] and inhibition of the mitochondrial permeability transition pore.[116]

Akt activation is a powerful survival signal that has been shown to mediate myocardial protection during late preconditioning and after reperfusion.[117] Akt is predominantly cytosolic and is activated through phosphorylation by insulin, insulin like growth factor-1, and also erythropoietin. Erythropoietin mediates the phosphorylation of Akt through phosphorylation of PDK$_1$ on activation of PI3K. Activated Akt can translocate to mitochondria, where it has been shown to exert beneficial effects including opening of mitochondrial K$_{ATP}$ channels,[117] activation of respiratory chain complexes and FoF1 ATPase,[118] and inhibition of the mitochondrial permeability transition pore.[119]

In support of a rapid erythropoietin protective effect, work in our laboratory in a rat model of cardiac arrest[71] and work in victims of out-of-hospital cardiac arrest in collaboration with Slovenian investigators[72] demonstrated the onset of hemodynamic benefits within minutes after erythropoietin administration. Both studies support the concept that erythropoietin facilitates return of spontaneous circulation by cell effects that result in the preservation of left ventricular myocardial distensibility, enabling preservation of left ventricular preload leading to hemodynamically more effective chest compression. Functionally, the effects are remarkably similar to the effects elicited by administration of NHE-1 inhibitors.[41,49]

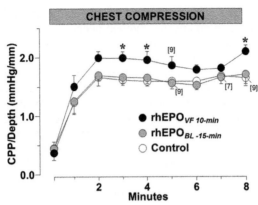

Fig. 11. Ratio between coronary pertusion pressure and depth of compression (CPP/Depth) during closed-chest resuscitation in rats treated with rhEPO at baseline (rhEPO$_{BL-15-min}$, n = 10; *shaded symbols*), during VF before starting chest compression (rhEPO$_{VF\ 10-min}$, n = 10; *closed symbols*), or with 0.9% NaCl (control, n = 10; *open symbols*). Numbers of rats remaining in VF and therefore receiving chest compression are indicated in brackets. Values are mean ± SEM. *$P<.05$ vs control by Dunnett's multicomparison method. (*Adapted from* Singh D, Kolarova JD, Wang S, et al. Myocardial protection by erythropoietin during resuscitation from ventricular fibrillation. Am J Ther 2007;14:361–8; with permission.)

Effects of erythropoietin during cardiac resuscitation

Studies in rats. The effects of erythropoietin for resuscitation were initially studied in a well-standardized rat model of electrically induced VF and closed-chest resuscitation using human recombinant erythropoietin (epoetin alfa, Amgen, Thousand Oaks, CA, USA).[71] Rats were subjected to a 10-minute interval of untreated VF followed by 8 minutes of closed-chest resuscitation (chest compression and ventilation with 100% oxygen) before defibrillation was attempted. Chest compression was adjusted to initially attain and subsequently maintain an aortic diastolic pressure between 26 and 28 mm Hg. Three groups of 10 rats each were randomized to receive a right atrial bolus of epoetin alfa (5000 IU/kg) at baseline 15 minutes before induction of VF (EPO$_{BL-15-min}$), at 10 minutes of VF before starting chest compression (EPO$_{VF\ 10-min}$), or to receive 0.9% NaCl solution (control) instead with the investigators blind to the treatment assignment.

Erythropoietin given coincident with the beginning of chest compression after 10 minutes of untreated VF—but not before induction of VF—promoted hemodynamically more effective chest compression such that the CPP/depth ratio averaged during the interval of chest compression was 25% higher in the group of rat that received erythropoietin at the beginning of chest compression. In **Fig. 11**, the CPP/depth ratio is depicted throughout chest compression. Post-resuscitation, EPO$_{VF\ 10-min}$ rats had significantly higher mean aortic pressure (**Fig. 12**) associated with numerically higher cardiac index and higher peripheral vascular resistance. The diminished effectiveness of erythropoietin when given before VF is intriguing and deserving of additional investigation.

Similar observations were made in a recent series of experiments in the same rat model of VF and closed-chest resuscitation described in the preceding text. In this series, hearts were removed after return of spontaneous circulation to examine in left ventricular tissue demonstrating activation of PKCε and Akt in both the cytosolic and the mitochondrial fractions.

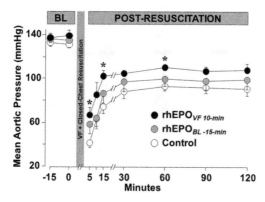

Fig. 12. Mean aortic pressure after return of spontaneous circulation in rats treated with rhEPO as described in **Fig. 11** and the text. BL, baseline. Values are mean ± SEM. *P<.05 vs control by Dunnett's multicomparison method. (*Adapted from* Singh D, Kolarova JD, Wang S, et al. Myocardial protection by erythropoietin during resuscitation from ventricular fibrillation. Am J Ther 2007;14:361–8; with permission.)

Studies in humans. A clinical study was performed in collaboration with Dr. Štefek Grmec, MD, PhD and the Maribor Emergency Medical Services (EMS) system in the city of Maribor and adjacent rural areas encompassing a population of approximately 200,000 inhabitants.[72] Resuscitation was attempted using regionally developed protocols that incorporate ILCOR 2005 recommendations. On arrival of the rescue squad an endotracheal tube was placed, verifying proper position by capnography. Positive pressure ventilation was provided with a tidal volume of ≈6 mL/kg delivered 10 times per minute unsynchronized to compressions. The rescue squad also established an intravenous access through an external vein within approximately 30 seconds. Patients assigned to erythropoietin received 90,000 IU of beta-epoetin (three vials of NeoRecormon 30,000 IU each, 1.8 mL total, Hoffman La Roche, Grenzacherstrasse, Basel, Switzerland) as a bolus dose within 1 or 2 minutes after start of chest compression followed by a 10-mL bolus of 0.9% NaCl. Beta-epoetin was kept refrigerated (2–8°C) in the ambulance until immediately before use. In every instance erythropoietin was given before any other drug.

By univariate analysis, administration of erythropoietin was associated with higher rates of admission to the receiving intensive care unit (ICU), return of spontaneous circulation (ROSC), 24-hour survival, and survival to hospital discharge when compared with concurrent controls and associated with higher rates of ICU admission, ROSC, and 24-hour survival when compared with matched controls after adjustment by multiple logistic regression for variables known to influence outcome (ie, age, male sex, witnessed arrest, time from call to start cardiopulmonary resuscitation [CPR], pulseless electrical activity, asystole, and bystander CPR). For comparison with concurrent controls, adjustment for these variables reduced the odds ratio but retained statistical significance for ICU admission and ROSC. For comparison with matched controls, adjustment increased the odds ratio, demonstrating statistical significance for all four outcomes (**Fig. 13**).

Based on our preceding work in rats, we hypothesized that erythropoietin—by preserving left ventricular myocardial distensibility—would prompt hemodynamically more effective chest compression and this effect would be reflected in a higher $P_{ET}CO_2$, which under low flow conditions is proportional to total and regional blood

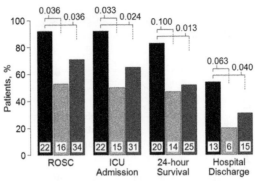

Fig. 13. Resuscitation and survival outcomes in patients who received erythropoietin (*black bars*, n − 24) compared with concurrent controls (*hatched bars*, n = 30) and with matched controls (*gray bars*, n = 48). Numbers inside bars denote patients for each outcome with the bar representing the percentage of the initial cohort. *P*-values were calculated by χ^2 test for each outcome adjusted by covariates with known predictive value (ie, age, male sex, witnessed arrest, time from call to start CPR, pulseless electrical activity, asystole, and bystander CPR) and are shown above bars. (*Data from* Grmec S, Strnad M, Kupnik D, et al. Erythropoietin facilitates the return of spontaneous circulation and survival in victims of out-of-hospital cardiac arrest. Resuscitation 2009;80:631–7.)

flow.[51,52] This was indeed the case. Victims who received erythropoietin had significantly higher $P_{ET}CO_2$ during chest compression (**Fig. 14**). Thus, these clinical observations—though based on a small sample size—are consistent with the hypothesis that erythropoietin, by preserving left ventricular myocardial distensibility, leads to hemodynamically more effective chest compression.

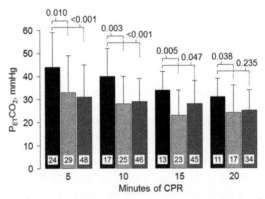

Fig. 14. End-tidal P_{CO_2} ($P_{ET}CO_2$) during cardiopulmonary resuscitation in patients who received erythropoietin (*black bars*, n = 24) compared with concurrent controls (*hatched bars*, n = 30) and with matched controls (*gray bars*, n = 48). Numbers inside bars denote patients remaining in cardiac arrest and receiving CPR. Data are presented as mean values with one standard deviation. *P*-values were calculated by unpaired *t*-test or by Mann–Whitney rank sum test for each time period and shown above bars. (*From* Grmec S, Strnad M, Kupnik D, et al. Erythropoietin facilitates the return of spontaneous circulation and survival in victims of out-of-hospital cardiac arrest. Resuscitation 2009;80:631–7; with permission.)

A total of six additional studies in cardiac arrest have been reported so far: four in rats[71,120–123] and one in humans.[124] In four of the animal studies, administration of erythropoietin before chest compression[71,123] or after restoration of spontaneous circulation[120,122] exerted beneficial myocardial effects, leading to preservation of left ventricular myocardial distensibility during chest compression[71] and less post-resuscitation myocardial dysfunction[71,120,122] with improved survival.[120,122,123] In the other animal study[121] and in the human study[124] the focus was on neurologic outcome. In the animal study, erythropoietin was given before cardiac arrest and showed no effects on neurologic recovery.

The human study was conducted in France by Cariou and colleagues.[124] This study enrolled a small group of patients who had suffered out-of-hospital cardiac arrest to examine possible neuroprotective effects of erythropoietin. In this study, five doses of 40,000 IU of EPO-alpha each were given over an interval of 48 hours to 18 patients who remained comatose—with a Glasgow Coma Scale of less than 7—after return of spontaneous circulation. It is important to emphasize that erythropoietin was given after ROSC and therefore in a setting of potential hemodynamic instability. The first dose of erythropoietin was given at a median time of 62 minutes (42–75, interquartile range [IQR]) after ROSC. The effects of erythropoietin were compared with 40 contemporaneous matched controls. There were differences favoring erythropoietin at 28 days in survival (55% vs 48%) and full neurological recovery (55% vs 38%), but the differences were statistically insignificant. The erythropoietin group experienced a high incidence of thrombocytosis (15% vs 5%), and one of these patients in the erythropoietin group suffered an occlusion of a coronary stent.

SUMMARY

The quest for interventions that could prevent or mitigate reperfusion injury has prompted an intense scientific pursuit for decades. This pursuit has broadened our understanding of the underlying pathogenic processes; yet, the development of clinical interventions targeting reperfusion injury has remained an elusive goal. Identification of functional intracellular effectors may lead to the recognition of more robust targets for therapeutic intervention. The growing evidence identifying mitochondria as effectors and targets of reperfusion injury is bringing renewed hope that novel and more effective interventions could be developed for resuscitation from cardiac arrest.

REFERENCES

1. Dong Z, Saikumar P, Weinberg JM, et al. Calcium in cell injury and death. Annu Rev Pathol 2006;1:405–34.
2. Halestrap AP. Calcium, mitochondria and reperfusion injury: a pore way to die. Biochem Soc Trans 2006;34(Pt 2):232–7.
3. Weisfeldt ML, Zweier J, Ambrosio G, et al. Evidence that free radicals result in reperfusion injury in heart muscle. Basic Life Sci 1988;49:911–9.
4. Vendelin M, Beraud N, Guerrero K, et al. Mitochondrial regular arrangement in muscle cells: a "crystal-like" pattern. Am J Physiol Cell Physiol 2005;288(3): C757–67.
5. Frezza C, Cipolat S, Martins de BO, et al. OPA1 controls apoptotic cristae remodeling independently from mitochondrial fusion. Cell 2006;126(1):177–89.
6. Mannella CA. The relevance of mitochondrial membrane topology to mitochondrial function. Biochim Biophys Acta 2006;1762(2):140–7.
7. Cai J, Yang J, Jones DP. Mitochondrial control of apoptosis: the role of cytochrome c. Biochim Biophys Acta 1998;1366(1-2):139–49.

8. Green DR, Reed JC. Mitochondria and apoptosis. Science 1998;281(5381): 1309–12.

9. Gao W, Pu Y, Luo KQ, et al. Temporal relationship between cytochrome *c* release and mitochondrial swelling during UV-induced apoptosis in living HeLa cells. J Cell Sci 2001;114(Pt 15):2855–62.

10. Bialik S, Cryns VL, Drincic A, et al. The mitochondrial apoptotic pathway is activated by serum and glucose deprivation in cardiac myocytes. Circ Res 1999;85(5):403–14.

11. Martinou I, Desagher S, Eskes R, et al. The release of cytochrome *c* from mitochondria during apoptosis of NGF-deprived sympathetic neurons is a reversible event. J Cell Biol 1999;144(5):883–9.

12. Charles I, Khalyfa A, Kumar DM, et al. Serum deprivation induces apoptotic cell death of transformed rat retinal ganglion cells via mitochondrial signaling pathways. Invest Ophthalmol Vis Sci 2005;46(4):1330–8.

13. Petrosillo G, Ruggiero FM, Pistolese M, et al. Ca^{2+}-induced reactive oxygen species production promotes cytochrome *c* release from rat liver mitochondria via mitochondrial permeability transition (MPT)-dependent and MPT-independent mechanisms: role of cardiolipin. J Biol Chem 2004;279(51):53103–8.

14. de Moissac D, Gurevich RM, Zheng H, et al. Caspase activation and mitochondrial cytochrome C release during hypoxia-mediated apoptosis of adult ventricular myocytes. J Mol Cell Cardiol 2000;32(1):53–63.

15. von Harsdorf R, Li PF, Dietz R. Signaling pathways in reactive oxygen species-induced cardiomyocyte apoptosis. Circulation 1999;99(22):2934–41.

16. Li P, Nijhawan D, Budihardjo I, et al. Cytochrome *c* and dATP-dependent formation of Apaf-1/caspase-9 complex initiates an apoptotic protease cascade. Cell 1997; 91(4):479–89.

17. Earnshaw WC, Martins LM, Kaufmann SH. Mammalian caspases: structure, activation, substrates, and functions during apoptosis. Annu Rev Biochem 1999;68:383–424.

18. Zou H, Li Y, Liu X, et al. An APAF-1.cytochrome *c* multimeric complex is a functional apoptosome that activates procaspase-9. J Biol Chem 1999;274(17):11549–56.

19. Radhakrishnan J, Wang S, Ayoub IM, et al. Circulating levels of cytochrome *c* after resuscitation from cardiac arrest: a marker of mitochondrial injury and predictor of survival. Am J Physiol Heart Circ Physiol 2007;292:H767–75.

20. Radhakrishnan J, Ayoub IM, Gazmuri RJ. Activation of caspase-3 may not contribute to postresuscitation myocardial dysfunction. Am J Physiol Heart Circ Physiol 2009;296(4):H1164–74.

21. Barczyk K, Kreuter M, Pryjma J, et al. Serum cytochrome *c* indicates in vivo apoptosis and can serve as a prognostic marker during cancer therapy. Int J Cancer 2005;116(2):167–73.

22. Renz A, Berdel WE, Kreuter M, et al. Rapid extracellular release of cytochrome *c* is specific for apoptosis and marks cell death in vivo. Blood 2001;98(5):1542–8.

23. Alleyne T, Joseph J, Sampson V. Cytochrome-*c* detection: a diagnostic marker for myocardial infarction. Appl Biochem Biotechnol 2001;90(2):97–105.

24. Adachi N, Hirota M, Hamaguchi M, et al. Serum cytochrome *c* level as a prognostic indicator in patients with systemic inflammatory response syndrome. Clin Chim Acta 2004;342(1-2):127–36.

25. Hosoya M, Nunoi H, Aoyama M, et al. Cytochrome c and tumor necrosis factor-alpha values in serum and cerebrospinal fluid of patients with influenza-associated encephalopathy. Pediatr Infect Dis J 2005;24(5):467–70.

26. Hosoya M, Kawasaki Y, Katayose M, et al. Prognostic predictive values of serum cytochrome *c*, cytokines, and other laboratory measurements in acute encephalopathy with multiple organ failure. Arch Dis Child 2006;91(6):469–72.

27. Crompton M. The mitochondrial permeability transition pore and its role in cell death. Biochem J 1999;341:233–49.

28. Halestrap AP. The mitochondrial permeability transition: its molecular mechanism and role in reperfusion injury. Biochem Soc Symp 1999;66:181–203.

29. Korsmeyer SJ, Wei MC, Saito M, et al. Pro-apoptotic cascade activates BID, which oligomerizes BAK or BAX into pores that result in the release of cytochrome c. Cell Death Differ 2000;7(12):1166–73.

30. Mikhailov V, Mikhailova M, Pulkrabek DJ, et al. Bcl-2 prevents Bax oligomerization in the mitochondrial outer membrane. J Biol Chem 2001;276(21):18361–74.

31. Lesnefsky EJ, Slabe TJ, Stoll MS, et al. Myocardial ischemia selectively depletes cardiolipin in rabbit heart subsarcolemmal mitochondria. Am J Physiol Heart Circ Physiol 2001;280(6):H2770–8.

32. Lesnefsky EJ, Chen Q, Slabe TJ, et al. Ischemia, rather than reperfusion, inhibits respiration through cytochrome oxidase in the isolated, perfused rabbit heart: role of cardiolipin. Am J Physiol Heart Circ Physiol 2004;287(1):H258–67.

33. Paradies G, Petrosillo G, Pistolese M, et al. Decrease in mitochondrial complex I activity in ischemic/reperfused rat heart: involvement of reactive oxygen species and cardiolipin. Circ Res 2004;94(1):53–9.

34. Binak K, Harmanci N, Sirmaci N, et al. Oxygen extraction rate of the myocardium at rest and on exercise in various conditions. Br Heart J 1967;29(3):422–7.

35. Yusa T, Obara S. Myocardial oxygen extraction rate under general anesthesia. Tohoku J Exp Med 1981;133(3):321–4.

36. Hoffman JIE. Maximal coronary flow and the concept of coronary vascular reserve. Circulation 1984;70:153–9.

37. Duggal C, Weil MH, Gazmuri RJ, et al. Regional blood flow during closed-chest cardiac resuscitation in rats. J Appl Physiol 1993;74:147–52.

38. Ditchey RV, Goto Y, Lindenfeld J. Myocardial oxygen requirements during experimental cardiopulmonary resuscitation. Cardiovasc Res 1992;26:791–7.

39. Gazmuri RJ, Berkowitz M, Cajigas H. Myocardial effects of ventricular fibrillation in the isolated rat heart. Crit Care Med 1999;27(8):1542–50.

40. Klouche K, Weil MH, Sun S, et al. Evolution of the stone heart after prolonged cardiac arrest. Chest 2002;122(3):1006–11.

41. Ayoub IM, Kolarova JD, Yi Z, et al. Sodium-hydrogen exchange inhibition during ventricular fibrillation: beneficial effects on ischemic contracture, action potential duration, reperfusion arrhythmias, myocardial function, and resuscitability. Circulation 2003;107:1804–9.

42. Cooley DA, Reul GJ, Wukasch DC. Ischemic contracture of the heart: "stone heart." Am J Cardiol 1972;29:575–7.

43. Katz AM, Tada M. The "stone heart": a challenge to the biochemist. Am J Cardiol 1972;29:578–80.

44. Sorrell VL, Altbach MI, Kern KB, et al. Images in cardiovascular medicine: continuous cardiac magnetic resonance imaging during untreated ventricular fibrillation. Circulation 2005;111(19):e294.

45. Koretsune Y, Marban E. Mechanism of ischemic contracture in ferret hearts: relative roles of [Ca2+]i elevation and ATP depletion. Am J Physiol 1990;258:H9–16.

46. Ayoub IM, Kolarova J, Kantola R, et al. Zoniporide preserves left ventricular compliance during ventricular fibrillation and minimizes post-resuscitation myocardial dysfunction through benefits on energy metabolism. Crit Care Med 2007;35:2329–36.

47. Gazmuri RJ. Effects of repetitive electrical shocks on postresuscitation myocardial function. Crit Care Med 2000;28(11 Suppl):N228–32.

48. Gazmuri RJ, Deshmukh S, Shah PR. Myocardial effects of repeated electrical defibrillations in the isolated fibrillating rat heart. Crit Care Med 2000;28:2690–6.

49. Kolarova JD, Ayoub IM, Gazmuri RJ. Cariporide enables hemodynamically more effective chest compression by leftward shift of its flow-depth relationship. Am J Physiol Heart Circ Physiol 2005;288:H2904–11.

50. Takino M, Okada Y. Firm myocardium in cardiopulmonary resuscitation. Resuscitation 1996;33:101–6.

51. Sanders AB, Atlas M, Ewy GA, et al. Expired PCO_2 as an index of coronary perfusion pressure. Am J Emerg Med 1985;3(2):147–9.

52. Gudipati CV, Weil MH, Bisera J, et al. Expired carbon dioxide: a noninvasive monitor of cardiopulmonary resuscitation. Circulation 1988;77:234–9.

53. Rubertsson S, Karlsten R. Increased cortical cerebral blood flow with LUCAS: a new device for mechanical chest compressions compared to standard external compressions during experimental cardiopulmonary resuscitation. Resuscitation 2005; 65(3):357–63.

54. van Alem AP, Post J, Koster RW. VF recurrence: characteristics and patient outcome in out-of-hospital cardiac arrest. Resuscitation 2003;59(2):181–8.

55. Gazmuri RJ, Weil MH, Bisera J, et al. Myocardial dysfunction after successful resuscitation from cardiac arrest. Crit Care Med 1996;24(6):992–1000.

56. Kern KB, Hilwig RW, Rhee KH, et al. Myocardial dysfunction after resuscitation from cardiac arrest: an example of global myocardial stunning. J Am Coll Cardiol 1996; 28:232–40.

57. Laurent I, Monchi M, Chiche JD, et al. Reversible myocardial dysfunction in survivors of out-of-hospital cardiac arrest. J Am Coll Cardiol 2002;40(12):2110–6.

58. Ruiz-Bailen M, Aguayo dH, Ruiz-Navarro S, et al. Reversible myocardial dysfunction after cardiopulmonary resuscitation. Resuscitation 2005;66(2):175–81.

59. Xu T, Tang W, Ristagno G, et al. Postresuscitation myocardial diastolic dysfunction following prolonged ventricular fibrillation and cardiopulmonary resuscitation. Crit Care Med 2008;36(1):188–92.

60. Hilwig RW, Berg RA, Kern KB, et al. Endothelin-1 vasoconstriction during swine cardiopulmonary resuscitation improves coronary perfusion pressures but worsens postresuscitation outcome. Circulation 2000;101(17):2097–102.

61. Kern KB, Hilwig RW, Berg RA, et al. Postresuscitation left ventricular systolic and diastolic dysfunction. Treatment with dobutamine. Circulation 1997;95(12):2610–3.

62. Vasquez A, Kern KB, Hilwig RW, et al. Optimal dosing of dobutamine for treating post-resuscitation left ventricular dysfunction. Resuscitation 2004;61(2):199–207.

63. Studer W, Wu X, Siegemund M, et al. Influence of dobutamine on the variables of systemic haemodynamics, metabolism, and intestinal perfusion after cardiopulmonary resuscitation in the rat. Resuscitation 2005;64(2):227–32.

64. Niemann JT, Garner D, Khaleeli E, et al. Milrinone facilitates resuscitation from cardiac arrest and attenuates postresuscitation myocardial dysfunction. Circulation 2003;108(24):3031–5.

65. Gazmuri RJ, Hoffner E, Kalcheim J, et al. Myocardial protection during ventricular fibrillation by reduction of proton-driven sarcolemmal sodium influx. J Lab Clin Med 2001;137(1):43–55.

66. Gazmuri RJ, Ayoub IM, Hoffner E, et al. Successful ventricular defibrillation by the selective sodium-hydrogen exchanger isoform-1 inhibitor cariporide. Circulation 2001;104:234–9.

67. Gazmuri RJ, Ayoub IM, Kolarova JD, et al. Myocardial protection during ventricular fibrillation by inhibition of the sodium-hydrogen exchanger isoform-1. Crit Care Med 2002;30(4 Suppl):S166–71.
68. Kolarova J, Yi Z, Ayoub IM, et al. Cariporide potentiates the effects of epinephrine and vasopressin by nonvascular mechanisms during closed-chest resuscitation. Chest 2005;127(4):1327–34.
69. Ayoub IM, Kolarova J, Kantola RL, et al. Cariporide minimizes adverse myocardial effects of epinephrine during resuscitation from ventricular fibrillation. Crit Care Med 2005;33(11):2599–605.
70. Wang S, Radhakrishnan J, Ayoub IM, et al. Limiting sarcolemmal Na^+ entry during resuscitation from VF prevents excess mitochondrial Ca^{2+} accumulation and attenuates myocardial injury. J Appl Physiol 2007;103:55–65.
71. Singh D, Kolarova JD, Wang S, et al. Myocardial protection by erythropoietin during resuscitation from ventricular fibrillation. Am J Ther 2007;14:361–8.
72. Grmec S, Strnad M, Kupnik D, et al. Erythropoietin facilitates the return of spontaneous circulation and survival in victims of out-of-hospital cardiac arrest. Resuscitation 2009;80:631–7.
73. von Planta M, Weil MH, Gazmuri RJ, et al. Myocardial acidosis associated with CO_2 production during cardiac arrest and resuscitation. Circulation 1989;80:684–92.
74. Kette F, Weil MH, Gazmuri RJ, et al. Intramyocardial hypercarbic acidosis during cardiac arrest and resuscitation. Crit Care Med 1993;21(6):901–6.
75. Noc M, Weil MH, Gazmuri RJ, et al. Ventricular fibrillation voltage as a monitor of the effectiveness of cardiopulmonary resuscitation. J Lab Clin Med 1994;124:421–6.
76. Karmazyn M, Sawyer M, Fliegel L. The Na(+)/H(+) exchanger: a target for cardiac therapeutic intervention. Curr Drug Targets Cardiovasc Haematol Disord 2005;5(4): 323–35.
77. Imahashi K, Kusuoka H, Hashimoto K, et al. Intracellular sodium accumulation during ischemia as the substrate for reperfusion injury. Circ Res 1999;84(12):1401–6.
78. Avkiran M, Ibuki C, Shimada Y, et al. Effects of acidic reperfusion on arrhythmias and Na(+)-K(+)-ATPase activity in regionally ischemic rat hearts. Am J Physiol 1996; 270(3 Pt 2):H957–64.
79. An J, Varadarajan SG, Camara A, et al. Blocking Na(+)/H(+) exchange reduces [Na(+)](i) and [Ca(2+)](i) load after ischemia and improves function in intact hearts. Am J Physiol 2001;281(6):H2398–2409.
80. Gunter TE, Buntinas L, Sparagna G, et al. Mitochondrial calcium transport: mechanisms and functions. Cell Calcium 2000;28(5–6):285–96.
81. Yamamoto S, Matsui K, Ohashi N. Protective effect of Na^+/H^+ exchange inhibitor, SM-20550, on impaired mitochondrial respiratory function and mitochondrial Ca^{2+} overload in ischemic/reperfused rat hearts. J Cardiovasc Pharmacol 2002;39(4): 569–75.
82. Borutaite V, Brown GC. Mitochondria in apoptosis of ischemic heart. FEBS Lett 2003;541(1–3):1–5.
83. Nasser FN, Walls JT, Edwards WD, et al. Lidocaine-induced reduction in size of experimental myocardial infarction. Am J Cardiol 1980;46(6):967–75.
84. Hinokiyama K, Hatori N, Ochi M, et al. Myocardial protective effect of lidocaine during experimental off-pump coronary artery bypass grafting. Ann Thorac Cardiovasc Surg 2003;9(1):36–42.
85. Ayoub IM, Radhakrishnan J, Gazmuri RJ. Targeting mitochondria for resuscitation from cardiac arrest. Crit Care Med 2008;36:S440–6.

86. Ayoub IM, Kolarova J, Gazmuri RJ. Cariporide given during resuscitation promotes return of electrically stable and mechanically competent cardiac activity. Resuscitation 2009;81:106–10.

87. Radhakrishnan J, Kolarova JD, Ayoub IM, et al. AVE4454B—a novel sodium-hydrogen exchanger isoform-1 inhibitor—compared less effective than cariporide for resuscitation from cardiac arrest. Translat Res 2011;157(2):71–80.

88. Paradis NA, Martin GB, Rivers EP, et al. Coronary perfusion pressure and the return of spontaneous circulation in human cardiopulmonary resuscitation. JAMA 1990; 263:1106–13.

89. Cai Z, Manalo DJ, Wei G, et al. Hearts from rodents exposed to intermittent hypoxia or erythropoietin are protected against ischemia-reperfusion injury. Circulation 2003; 108(1):79–85.

90. Calvillo L, Latini R, Kajstura J, et al. Recombinant human erythropoietin protects the myocardium from ischemia-reperfusion injury and promotes beneficial remodeling. Proc Natl Acad Sci USA 2003;100(8):4802–6.

91. Moon C, Krawczyk M, Ahn D, et al. Erythropoietin reduces myocardial infarction and left ventricular functional decline after coronary artery ligation in rats. Proc Natl Acad Sci USA 2003;100(20):11612–7.

92. Parsa CJ, Matsumoto A, Kim J, et al. A novel protective effect of erythropoietin in the infarcted heart. J Clin Invest 2003;112(7):999–1007.

93. Tramontano AF, Muniyappa R, Black AD, et al. Erythropoietin protects cardiac myocytes from hypoxia-induced apoptosis through an Akt-dependent pathway. Biochem Biophys Res Commun 2003;308(4):990–4.

94. Cai Z, Semenza GL. Phosphatidylinositol-3-kinase signaling is required for erythropoietin-mediated acute protection against myocardial ischemia/reperfusion injury. Circulation 2004;109(17):2050–3.

95. Lipsic E, van der MP, Henning RH, et al. Timing of erythropoietin treatment for cardioprotection in ischemia/reperfusion. J Cardiovasc Pharmacol 2004;44(4): 473–9.

96. Parsa CJ, Kim J, Riel RU, et al. Cardioprotective effects of erythropoietin in the reperfused ischemic heart: a potential role for cardiac fibroblasts. J Biol Chem 2004;279(20):20655–62.

97. Wright GL, Hanlon P, Amin K, et al. Erythropoietin receptor expression in adult rat cardiomyocytes is associated with an acute cardioprotective effect for recombinant erythropoietin during ischemia-reperfusion injury. FASEB J 2004;18(9):1031–3.

98. Namiuchi S, Kagaya Y, Ohta J, et al. High serum erythropoietin level is associated with smaller infarct size in patients with acute myocardial infarction who undergo successful primary percutaneous coronary intervention. J Am Coll Cardiol 2005; 45(9):1406–12.

99. Brines ML, Ghezzi P, Keenan S, et al. Erythropoietin crosses the blood–brain barrier to protect against experimental brain injury. Proc Natl Acad Sci USA 2000;97(19): 10526–31.

100. Siren AL, Fratelli M, Brines M, et al. Erythropoietin prevents neuronal apoptosis after cerebral ischemia and metabolic stress. Proc Natl Acad Sci USA 2001;98(7): 4044–9.

101. Ruscher K, Freyer D, Karsch M, et al. Erythropoietin is a paracrine mediator of ischemic tolerance in the brain: evidence from an in vitro model. J Neurosci 2002;22(23):10291–301.

102. Ghezzi P, Brines M. Erythropoietin as an antiapoptotic, tissue-protective cytokine. Cell Death Differ 2004;11:S37–44.

103. Celik M, Gokmen N, Erbayraktar S, et al. Erythropoietin prevents motor neuron apoptosis and neurologic disability in experimental spinal cord ischemic injury. Proc Natl Acad Sci USA 2002;99(4):2258–63.

104. Vesey DA, Cheung C, Pat B, et al. Erythropoietin protects against ischaemic acute renal injury. Nephrol Dial Transplant 2004;19(2):348–55.

105. Abdelrahman M, Sharples EJ, McDonald MC, et al. Erythropoietin attenuates the tissue injury associated with hemorrhagic shock and myocardial ischemia. Shock 2004;22(1):63–9.

106. Buemi M, Vaccaro M, Sturiale A, et al. Recombinant human erythropoietin influences revascularization and healing in a rat model of random ischaemic flaps. Acta Derm Venereol 2002;82(6):411–7.

107. Rui T, Feng Q, Lei M, et al. Erythropoietin prevents the acute myocardial inflammatory response induced by ischemia/reperfusion via induction of AP-1. Cardiovasc Res 2005;65(3):719–27.

108. Li Y, Takemura G, Okada H, et al. Reduction of inflammatory cytokine expression and oxidative damage by erythropoietin in chronic heart failure. Cardiovasc Res 2006;71(4):684–94.

109. van der MP, Lipsic E, Henning RH, et al. Erythropoietin induces neovascularization and improves cardiac function in rats with heart failure after myocardial infarction. J Am Coll Cardiol 2005;46(1):125–33.

110. Hirata A, Minamino T, Asanuma H, et al. Erythropoietin enhances neovascularization of ischemic myocardium and improves left ventricular dysfunction after myocardial infarction in dogs. J Am Coll Cardiol 2006;48(1):176–84.

111. Holmuhamedov EL, Jovanovic S, Dzeja PP, et al. Mitochondrial ATP-sensitive K^+ channels modulate cardiac mitochondrial function. Am J Physiol 1998;275(5 Pt 2):H1567–76.

112. Wald M, Gutnisky A, Borda E, et al. Erythropoietin modified the cardiac action of ouabain in chronically anaemic-uraemic rats. Nephron 1995;71(2):190–6.

113. Liu H, Zhang HY, Zhu X, et al. Preconditioning blocks cardiocyte apoptosis: role of K(ATP) channels and PKC-epsilon. Am J Physiol 2002;282(4):H1380–6.

114. Guo D, Nguyen T, Ogbi M, et al. Protein kinase C-epsilon coimmunoprecipitates with cytochrome oxidase subunit IV and is associated with improved cytochrome-c oxidase activity and cardioprotection. Am J Physiol Heart Circ Physiol 2007;293(4): H2219–30.

115. Chen CH, Budas GR, Churchill EN, et al. Activation of aldehyde dehydrogenase-2 reduces ischemic damage to the heart. Science 2008;321(5895):1493–5.

116. Baines CP, Song CX, Zheng YT, et al. Protein kinase Cepsilon interacts with and inhibits the permeability transition pore in cardiac mitochondria. Circ Res 2003;92(8): 873–80.

117. Ahmad N, Wang Y, Haider KH, et al. Cardiac protection by mitoKATP channels is dependent on Akt translocation from cytosol to mitochondria during late preconditioning. Am J Physiol Heart Circ Physiol 2006;290(6):H2402–8.

118. Shaik ZP, Fifer EK, Nowak G. Akt activation improves oxidative phosphorylation in renal proximal tubular cells following nephrotoxicant injury. Am J Physiol Renal Physiol 2008;294(2):F423–32.

119. Kobayashi H, Miura T, Ishida H, et al. Limitation of infarct size by erythropoietin is associated with translocation of Akt to the mitochondria after reperfusion. Clin Exp Pharmacol Physiol 2008;35(7):812–9.

120. Huang CH, Hsu CY, Chen HW, et al. Erythropoietin improves postresuscitation myocardial dysfunction and survival in the asphyxia-induced cardiac arrest model. Shock 2007;28(1):53–8.

121. Popp E, Vogel P, Teschendorf P, et al. Effects of the application of erythropoietin on cerebral recovery after cardiac arrest in rats. Resuscitation 2007;74(2):344–51.

122. Huang CH, Hsu CY, Tsai MS, et al. Cardioprotective effects of erythropoietin on postresuscitation myocardial dysfunction in appropriate therapeutic windows. Crit Care Med 2008;36:S467–73.

123. Incagnoli P, Ramond A, Joyeux-Faure M, et al. Erythropoietin improved initial resuscitation and increased survival after cardiac arrest in rats. Resuscitation 2009; 80(6):696–700.

124. Cariou A, Claessens YE, Pene F, et al. Early high-dose erythropoietin therapy and hypothermia after out-of-hospital cardiac arrest: a matched control study. Resuscitation 2008;76(3):397–404.

Advances in Brain Resuscitation: Beyond Hypothermia

Matthias Derwall, MD[a],*, Michael Fries, MD, PhD[b]

KEYWORDS
- Xenon • Induced hypothermia • Cardiac arrest
- Cardiopulmonary resuscitation • Cerebral ischemia

Less than a third of all successfully resuscitated patients with out-of-hospital cardiac arrest (OHCA) survive until hospital discharge despite significant advances in primary and intensive care treatment in recent years.[1,2] The so-called post cardiac arrest syndrome, which predominantly affects heart and brain, is responsible for the high mortality rate among OHCA patients.[3] Several new therapeutic approaches aiming at this condition have been conceived of and tested in the last decade, including the use of mild therapeutic hypothermia (MTH), volatile anesthetics, and extracorporeal cardiovascular assist devices. Whereas most of these approaches remain experimental, some are under scrutiny with the aim of being implemented into clinical practice. However, MTH still represents the current gold standard in postarrest care.

This review article gives an overview of established strategies and protocols while depicting current developments in the fight against neurologic sequelae following cardiac arrest.

THERAPEUTIC HYPOTHERMIA

The neuroprotective effects of induced hypothermia have been described in modern medicine since the early 1960s, when intraoperative cooling was first introduced into neurosurgery to prevent cerebral sequelae caused by temporary ischemia.[4] The early use of induced hypothermia included target body temperatures below 30°C, which are associated with cardiac arrhythmias, coagulopathy, and elevated infection rates. To reduce these adverse side effects, studies at the beginning of the last century

For this article, no industrial financial support was received.

The Department of Anesthesiology has received funding from Messer-Griesheim GmbH, Business Unit Messer Medical, Krefeld, Germany, and Air Liquide, Paris, France.

[a] Department of Anesthesiology, University Hospital Rheinisch-Westfälische Technische Hochschule Aachen, Pauwelsstr, 30, D-52074, Aachen, Germany
[b] Department of Surgical Intensive Care, University Hospital Rheinisch-Westfälische Technische Hochschule Aachen, Pauwelsstr, 30, D-52074, Aachen, Germany
* Corresponding author.

E-mail address: mderwall@ukaachen.de

Crit Care Clin 28 (2012) 271–281
doi:10.1016/j.ccc.2011.10.010
0749-0704/12/$ – see front matter © 2012 Elsevier Inc. All rights reserved.

focused on the efficacy of lowering body temperature to around $33 \pm 1°C$ following successful resuscitation, now widely referred to as mild therapeutic hypothermia.[5,6] Promising results from animal studies[7-10] and the landmark Hypothermia After Cardiac Arrest trial[5] finally led to the introduction of MTH into international resuscitation guidelines in 2005.[11] At its first appearance in the 2005 guidelines, MTH was recommended only for unconscious adult patients with spontaneous circulation after OHCA, when the initial rhythm was ventricular fibrillation (VF).[11] Current recommendations suggest consideration of induced hypothermia for comatose adult patients with return of spontaneous circulation (ROSC) after in-hospital cardiac arrest of any initial rhythm or after OHCA with an initial rhythm of pulseless electric activity or asystole.[12] With only 6 patients requiring treatment to save 1 additional life, MTH is the single most effective intervention and therefore the gold standard in postresuscitation care today.[13]

Therapeutic hypothermia had long been thought to unfold its cytoprotective properties simply via unspecific inhibition of catabolic processes throughout the organism during the reperfusion period. While this aspect is still true, other mechanisms involved in neuroprotection following global ischemia have been revealed recently. These mechanisms are particularly interesting because they are not only important for understanding the processes involved but might also be used as targets for other therapeutic agents to augment the efficacy of MTH in the future. For instance, MTH is known to induce a decrease in brain glycine and p53 protein levels[14,15] Furthermore, MTH blocks delta-protein kinase C and several other proteins that induce apoptotic cell death, including those from the Bcl-2 family.[16,17] The noble gas xenon in particular has been found to have a considerable effect on these targets, making it one possible candidate to augment MTH potency.

Although the beneficial effects of MTH following cardiac arrest are well-described and mutually accepted today, it remains controversial how, when, and for how long to cool. One controversy during the wake of the introduction of MTH into guidelines in 2005 was whether intravascular cooling devices are superior to surface cooling using simple measures such as ice bags or cooling blankets. Although the intravascular devices do have their benefits with regard to maintaining target temperature over time,[18] they come with certain disadvantages because of their invasiveness and higher costs.[19] Time until reaching target temperature, now considered to be the most important parameter in MTH therapy, is shorter using conventional surface-cooling techniques.[18] Furthermore, the more precise cooling with intravascular devices does not seem to be associated with a better neurologic outcome or long-term survival.[20] Therefore, surface cooling, which can be easily achieved at a very low price with simple measures such as ice water–filled bags, seems to be equally effective.

A novel development was the introduction of targeted cooling of cerebral structures instead of whole body cooling. Targeted cooling has been shown to gain effectiveness similar to whole body cooling while reducing nursing efforts during MTH.[21] Coupled with the paradigm that cooling of the patient should occur as soon as possible following ROSC, the idea of isolated cerebral cooling led to the development of an intranasal cooling device[22-24] that can be easily applied by nonphysician emergency medical personnel during the resuscitation procedure. The device takes advantage of the close proximity of the nasal cavity to cerebral structures and applies a perfluorocarbon directly into the nasal cavity, which cools the surface because of evaporation. Before ROSC, cerebral structures are cooled through direct conduction. Upon return of circulation, the brain and body are cooled through indirect convection because the cooled circulating blood removes heat via the bloodstream. The advantage of this system is the rapid onset of cooling combined with a quick and easy application that can be performed without hindering chest compressions or access to the airway.[22] In the PRINCE (Pre-ROSC Intranasal Cooling Effectiveness) study published in 2011, this device proved to be significantly faster for regional and systemic cooling compared with conventional surface cooling.[25] It is yet to be proved whether this novel approach of shifting cooling into the prehospital setting and accelerating the cooling process will translate into better ROSC and long-term neurologic outcome parameters.

MEDICAL GASES

Several studies identified neuronal excitotoxicity caused by overactivation of N-methyl-D-aspartate (NMDA) glutamate receptors as one of the primordial neuropathologic processes in hypoxic-ischemic neuronal injury.[26,27] However, several clinical trials have failed to translate this knowledge into clinical practice, in some cases because of a lack in efficacy and in others due to adverse side effects of the agents tested.[28–30] Remarkable exemptions to these results are findings from animal studies using medical gases such as isoflurane,[31] xenon,[32] helium,[33] and argon.[34]. Xenon not only provides neuroprotective effects, it also seems to act in a synergistic pattern with therapeutic hypothermia.[35-38] Whereas xenon's neuroprotective properties could be associated with several molecular targets including the NMDA receptor and its impact on intracellular calcium homeostasis,[39] it is still unclear whether other noble gases with similar properties such as helium[33] and argon[34] act via equivalent pathways or through other unknown mechanisms. Dickinson and colleagues[40] showed by using grand canonical Monte Carlo simulations that xenon and isoflurane share the same binding site on the NMDA receptor, explaining in part the neuroprotective and anesthetic effects shared by both gases.

Xenon, although colorless and odorless and considered to be chemically inert, does interact with various biological systems.[39] Inhaled concentrations of more than 40% cause rapid onset of unconsciousness that has been shown to be mediated by xenon's ability to inhibit the NMDA receptor in the central nervous system (CNS).[41] Xenon seems to share some of the mechanisms involved in MTH-mediated neuroprotection,[36,42] like inducing a decrease in cerebral glycine and p53 protein levels[14,15] or proapoptotic proteins such as those from the Bcl-2 family.[16,17] Furthermore, Xenon provides additional protection by activating the 2-pore domain potassium channel and by effectively opening the adenosine triphosphate–dependent potassium channel.[43,44]

Xenon's organ-protective properties have been shown in several models of neurologic injury including stroke, traumatic brain injury, and hypoxic-ischemic encephalopathy.[45–50] Inhaled xenon improved functional recovery in a porcine model of cardiac arrest and significantly reduced neuronal damage when given 1 hour after successful resuscitation.[32] Xenon may also be effective within a prolonged time frame after ROSC, ranging from 10 minutes[51] up to 5 hours.[32] Accumulating data from several experiments in rodents revealed a potential synergistic effect of MTH and xenon, resulting in a significantly greater degree of protection than achieved with either of the interventions alone.[35–38] Unpublished data from the authors' group demonstrate that the combined short-term administration of xenon in addition to MTH is superior to MTH alone in terms of a significant neurocognitive recovery in a large animal model of prolonged cardiac arrest and resuscitation in pigs. This study furthermore revealed a preserved hemodynamic stability in the early postresuscitation period when xenon was given during the induction of therapeutic hypothermia. These results confirm findings from other animal models, for instance the works of Chakkarapani and colleagues[52] who demonstrated in a pediatric model of hypoxic-ischemic encephalopathy that the combined administration of these two interventions yields a greater functional recovery than xenon or MTH alone.

Notably, xenon was only administered for a short 1-hour period in the authors' investigation, but it still yielded a significant improvement of MTH's neuroprotective properties. This observation is particularly interesting because due to its rarity xenon is costly, which will probably preclude its widespread clinical use, at least as an anesthetic.[39]

Xenon's cytoprotective properties are not limited to cerebral tissues. Although knowledge of xenon's neuroprotective effects is primarily based on data from animal experiments, xenon's effects on cardiac function have been extensively investigated not only in various animal models[53–55] but also in clinical trials, in which xenon proved to preserve arterial pressures and heart rate variability in hemodynamically unstable patients.[56–58] In healthy patients, xenon has been proved a safe anesthetic with rapid recovery characteristics and only minor side effects on hemodynamics.[58,59] Xenon's minimal impact on hemodynamic stability may also be particularly desirable for patients recovering from cardiac arrest, because cardiac arrhythmias often occur as a manifestation of myocardial infarction and patients successfully resuscitated from OHCA exhibit left ventricular dysfunction as a result of myocardial stunning.[60,61] Hence, xenon may offer advantages over other neuroprotective gases such as isoflurane during the postresuscitation period.

Currently, a phase II clinical trial has been deployed at the authors' center. The trial is is going to explore the efficacy of MTH combined with xenon in OHCA (ClinicalTrials.gov Identifier NCT01262729). Similar trials are currently investigating the combination of xenon and MTH in this setting (NCT00879892) and also following perinatal asphyxia (NCT00934700).

INTRAVASCULAR RESUSCITATION

Recently, the cardiopulmonary resuscitation (CPR) procedure itself has received considerable attention in terms of periarrest care. Because it is well-known that conventional chest compressions only account for 20% to 30% of baseline cardiac output and postarrest hemodynamics are characterized by postresuscitation myocardial dysfunction, several groups are testing supportive devices for improving myocardial and cerebral perfusion during and after CPR. Data from patients suffering from in-hospital cardiac arrest revealed that circulatory support from an extracorporeal membrane oxygenator can improve the clinical outcome by optimizing periarrest hemodynamics.[62] Other approaches to optimize periarrest hemodynamics with less invasive measures include intravascular devices that are advanced percutaneously into the left ventricle.

The paradigm shift in neuroprotection from postarrest to intraarrest measures is due to a reappraisal of long-established knowledge of cellular physiology. Because the CNS does not contain comprehensive amounts of oxygen or glucose, its tissues rely solely on a permanent supply via the circulation. Therefore, the CNS can only compensate a suspension of blood flow for 4 to 8 seconds without any alterations in its physiologic parameters. After 15 to 30 seconds individuals lose consciousness; after 7 to 15 minutes, resuscitation efforts for the brain are futile in most cases.[63] The lack of global perfusion during cardiac arrest leads via a cascade of diverse mechanisms to systemic organ dysfunction or failure, depending on the organ's individual susceptibility to ischemia-reperfusion injury. Cardiac dysfunction following cardiac arrest is frequently observed and often results in left ventricular pump failure. The severity of this postresuscitation myocardial dysfunction correlates not only with the duration of ischemia but also with the number of defibrillation attempts and amount of energy applied to the myocardium.[60,61] It is obvious that optimizing the circulation during CPR by supporting or replacing cardiac function during and after CPR is the single most important action to improve brain resuscitation and therefore the patient's prognosis. To achieve this goal, recent CPR guidelines have focused again on the importance of chest compressions[64] instead of early defibrillation, which had been advocated before.[65]

However, it is well-known that conventional chest compressions can only account for about 30% of baseline cardiac output, even under ideal conditions.[66] It is likely that the generated blood flow during CPR will be considerably lower in clinical reality, because responders frequently work under difficult conditions and often overestimate their ability to provide sufficient chest compressions in self-assessment studies.[67]

Technical means to support or replace cardiac function such as extracorporeal membrane oxygenation (ECMO) are very invasive and are only feasible under certain circumstances. Furthermore, these means frequently require a surgical procedure to introduce large-bore catheters into jugular or femoral vessels.[68] In addition, ECMO poses risk for traumatic hemolysis and adverse dead space effects during priming of the system. CPR support via ECMO (eCPR) also requires chest compressions and profound anticoagulation because of extensive foreign surfaces of tubing and oxygenator, which may not be possible in all cardiac arrest patients. Despite its invasive character, eCPR has been shown in a single-center clinical trial to improve 1-year survival in patients suffering in-hospital cardiac arrest as compared with conventional chest compressions alone.[62]

An alternative, less invasive device has recently been proposed for use in the setting of cardiac arrest and CPR. The Impella 2.5 percutaneous left ventricular assist device (LVAD) is able to pump 2.5 L/min through a miniature turbine at the tip of a 12F catheter, translating into up to 74% of restored baseline cardiac output. For this purpose the LVAD is introduced via a 13F sheath introducer into the femoral artery and advanced into the left ventricle. While blood is sucked in at the tip of the catheter, the outflow tract is situated only a few inches proximal to the tip, behind the aortic valve. Originally designed as a bridging device for cardiac failure, the device releases the ventricle from filling pressure and improves perfusion of the coronary arteries and the brain. Its use in the setting of cardiac arrest and CPR has recently been described in two case reports[69,70] and tested in three animal studies.[71–73] These animal studies revealed that the LVAD is capable of restoring up to 74% of baseline myocardial and up to 65% of cerebral perfusion during VF.[73] The maintenance of cerebral blood flow by the LVAD during VF prevented serum markers of cerebral ischemia from rising during 20 minutes of VF. After 40 minutes of VF, lactate was the only marker to be significantly elevated in the same investigation.[71]

Furthermore, the same group compared the efficacy of the LVAD versus cardiac massage in an open-chest model of cardiac arrest.[72] In this study, the LVAD was equal or superior to manual compressions in terms of organ perfusion and rates of successful defibrillation after 20 minutes of VF.

The novel concept of intravascular resuscitation has proved to significantly augment hemodynamics during CPR but has yet to show whether this improvement translates into a higher rate of successful ROSC and finally into better neurocognitive outcomes. Finally, it needs to be shown whether use of these devices in the field can be feasible and effective.

CONCEPTS BEYOND HYPOTHERMIA, GASES, AND HEMODYNAMICS

Beyond the concepts of therapeutic hypothermia, medical gases, and optimizing periarrest hemodynamics, other neuroprotective strategies have been proposed in recent years. Whereas some concepts have been thoroughly investigated but soon abolished because of disappointing results, others seem to be promising but still lacking sufficient data to be thoroughly understood and appreciated. Two of these declining or emerging strategies are worth mentioning.

The swamp gas hydrogen sulfide (H_2S) or donor compounds like sodium sulfide showed astonishing effects in rodents; the inhalation of very low doses led to a hibernation-like state[74] in which mice were protected from asphyxia.[75] With the idea that infusion or inhalation of H_2S would help to buy time in the chain of survival,[76] several investigators initiated studies using H_2S in diverse animal models of hypoxia/ischemia. Whereas several investigators described improvements in small animal models of hemorrhagic shock[77] or CPR,[78] others showed that these results may not be easily transferable to large mammals.[68,79] Although H_2S remains an interesting compound with unanticipated roles in physiology,[80,81] its significance as a neuroprotective agent is less clear at this time.

The cytoprotective effects of erythropoietin (EPO) seem to be independent of EPO's erythropoietic and neovascularization properties and have first been described in myocardial ischemia-reperfusion injury.[82,83] Although there are only limited data on EPO's neuroprotective properties from animal studies, some intriguing small-scale clinical trials have shed light on this novel drug in periarrest care.[84,85] These studies not only showed benefits in initial ROSC rates but also affected survival to hospital discharge in the EPO groups. Further studies focusing on long-term survival, neurocognitive outcome, and setups within large clinical trials (NCT00999583) will have to prove whether this novel treatment may become a new standard in postarrest care.

SUMMARY

Preserving the brain from ischemia-reperfusion injury is the main challenge of resuscitation research today. Whereas several promising medical gases are about to expand the neuroprotective care after ROSC, new technical devices are emerging that may be the next leap forward in CPR and brain resuscitation. With optimizing postarrest hemodynamics during and after CPR, they may help not only to yield higher rates of ROSC but also to help more patients survive until hospital discharge and finally profit in terms of a better neurocognitive outcome and long-term quality of life. Until then, MTH will remain the gold standard in brain resuscitation, eventually expanded by novel technical devices for prehospital targeted cooling of the brain.

REFERENCES

1. Nolan J, Laver S. Outcome of out-of-hospital cardiac arrest. Anaesthesia 2007; 62(10):1082–3 [author reply: 1083].
2. Olasveengen TM, Sunde K, Brunborg C, et al. Intravenous drug administration during out-of-hospital cardiac arrest: a randomized trial. JAMA 2009;302(20):2222–9.
3. Neumar RW, Nolan JP, Adrie C, et al. Post-cardiac arrest syndrome: epidemiology, pathophysiology, treatment, and prognostication. A consensus statement from the International Liaison Committee on Resuscitation (American Heart Association, Australian and New Zealand Council on Resuscitation, European Resuscitation Council, Heart and Stroke Foundation of Canada, InterAmerican Heart Foundation, Resuscitation Council of Asia, and the Resuscitation Council of Southern Africa); the American Heart Association Emergency Cardiovascular Care Committee; the Council on Cardiovascular Surgery and Anesthesia; the Council on Cardiopulmonary, Perioperative, and Critical Care; the Council on Clinical Cardiology; and the Stroke Council. Circulation 2008;118(23):2452–83.
4. Woodhall B, Sealy WC, Hall KD, et al. Craniotomy under conditions of quinidine-protected cardioplegia and profound hypothermia. Ann Surg 1960;152:37–44.
5. Hypothermia After Cardiac Arrest Study Group. Mild therapeutic hypothermia to improve the neurologic outcome after cardiac arrest. N Engl J Med 2002;346(8): 549–56.
6. Bernard SA, Gray TW, Buist MD, et al. Treatment of comatose survivors of out-of-hospital cardiac arrest with induced hypothermia. N Engl J Med 2002;346(8):557–63.

7. Abella BS, Zhao D, Alvarado J, et al. Intra-arrest cooling improves outcomes in a murine cardiac arrest model. Circulation 2004;109(22):2786–91.
8. Katz LM, Young A, Frank JE, et al. Neurotensin-induced hypothermia improves neurologic outcome after hypoxic-ischemia. Crit Care Med 2004;32(3):806–10.
9. Sterz F, Safar P, Tisherman S, et al. Mild hypothermic cardiopulmonary resuscitation improves outcome after prolonged cardiac arrest in dogs. Crit Care Med 1991;19(3):379–89.
10. Xiao F, Safar P, Radovsky A. Mild protective and resuscitative hypothermia for asphyxial cardiac arrest in rats. Am J Emerg Med 1998;16(1):17–25.
11. 2005 International Consensus on Cardiopulmonary Resuscitation and Emergency Cardiovascular Care Science with Treatment Recommendations. Part 4: advanced life support. Resuscitation 2005;67(2-3):213–47.
12. Peberdy MA, Callaway CW, Neumar RW, et al. Part 9: post-cardiac arrest care: 2010 American Heart Association Guidelines for Cardiopulmonary Resuscitation and Emergency Cardiovascular Care. Circulation 2010;122(18 Suppl 3):S768–86.
13. Holzer M, Bernard SA, Hachimi-Idrissi S, et al. Hypothermia for neuroprotection after cardiac arrest: systematic review and individual patient data meta-analysis. Crit Care Med 2005;33(2):414–8.
14. Ji X, Luo Y, Ling F, et al. Mild hypothermia diminishes oxidative DNA damage and pro-death signaling events after cerebral ischemia: a mechanism for neuroprotection. Front Biosci 2007;12:1737–47.
15. Ooboshi H, Ibayashi S, Takano K, et al. Hypothermia inhibits ischemia-induced efflux of amino acids and neuronal damage in the hippocampus of aged rats. Brain Res 2000;884(1-2):23–30.
16. Schmitt KR, Diestel A, Lehnardt S, et al. Hypothermia suppresses inflammation via ERK signaling pathway in stimulated microglial cells. J Neuroimmunol 2007;189(1-2):7–16.
17. Zhao H, Yenari MA, Sapolsky RM, et al. Mild postischemic hypothermia prolongs the time window for gene therapy by inhibiting cytochrome C release. Stroke 2004;35(2):572–7.
18. Finley Caulfield A, Rachabattula S, Eyngorn I, et al. A comparison of cooling techniques to treat cardiac arrest patients with hypothermia. Stroke Res Treat 2011;2011: 690506.
19. Nielsen N, Sunde K, Hovdenes J, et al. Adverse events and their relation to mortality in out-of-hospital cardiac arrest patients treated with therapeutic hypothermia. Crit Care Med 2011;39(1):57–64.
20. Tomte O, Draegni T, Mangschau A, et al. A comparison of intravascular and surface cooling techniques in comatose cardiac arrest survivors. Crit Care Med 2011;39(3):443–9.
21. Tsai MS, Barbut D, Tang W, et al. Rapid head cooling initiated coincident with cardiopulmonary resuscitation improves success of defibrillation and post-resuscitation myocardial function in a porcine model of prolonged cardiac arrest. J Am Coll Cardiol 2008;51(20):1988–90.
22. Busch HJ, Eichwede F, Fodisch M, et al. Safety and feasibility of nasopharyngeal evaporative cooling in the emergency department setting in survivors of cardiac arrest. Resuscitation 2010;81(8):943–9.
23. Wang H, Barbut D, Tsai MS, et al. Intra-arrest selective brain cooling improves success of resuscitation in a porcine model of prolonged cardiac arrest. Resuscitation 2010;81(5):617–21.
24. Yu T, Barbut D, Ristagno G, et al. Survival and neurological outcomes after nasopharyngeal cooling or peripheral vein cold saline infusion initiated during cardiopulmonary resuscitation in a porcine model of prolonged cardiac arrest. Crit Care Med 2010; 38(3):916–21.

25. Castren M, Nordberg P, Svensson L, et al. Intra-arrest transnasal evaporative cooling: a randomized, prehospital, multicenter study (PRINCE: Pre-ROSC IntraNasal Cooling Effectiveness). Circulation 2011;122(7):729–36.

26. Choi KT, Chung JK, Kwak CS, et al. Effect of hypocapnia on extracellular glutamate and glycine concentrations during peri-ischemic period in the rabbit hippocampus. J Korean Med Sci 1994;9(5):394–401.

27. Lipton P. Ischemic cell death in brain neurons. Physiol Rev 1999;79(4):1431–568.

28. Ikonomidou C, Turski L. Why did NMDA receptor antagonists fail clinical trials for stroke and traumatic brain injury? Lancet Neurol 2002;1(6):383–6.

29. Kemp JA, McKernan RM. NMDA receptor pathways as drug targets. Nat Neurosci 2002;(5 Suppl):1039–42.

30. Lee JM, Zipfel GJ, Choi DW. The changing landscape of ischaemic brain injury mechanisms. Nature 1999;399(6738 Suppl):A7–14.

31. Derwall M, Timper A, Kottmann K, et al. Neuroprotective effects of the inhalational anesthetics isoflurane and xenon after cardiac arrest in pigs. Crit Care Med 2008; 36(11 Suppl):S492–5.

32. Fries M, Nolte KW, Coburn M, et al. Xenon reduces neurohistopathological damage and improves the early neurological deficit after cardiac arrest in pigs. Crit Care Med 2008;36(8):2420–6.

33. Jawad N, Rizvi M, Gu J, et al. Neuroprotection (and lack of neuroprotection) afforded by a series of noble gases in an in vitro model of neuronal injury. Neurosci Lett 2009;460(3):232–6.

34. Loetscher PD, Rossaint J, Rossaint R, et al. Argon: neuroprotection in in vitro models of cerebral ischemia and traumatic brain injury. Crit Care 2009;13(6):R206.

35. Hobbs C, Thoresen M, Tucker A, et al. Xenon and hypothermia combine additively, offering long-term functional and histopathologic neuroprotection after neonatal hypoxia/ischemia. Stroke 2008;39(4):1307–13.

36. Ma D, Hossain M, Chow A, et al. Xenon and hypothermia combine to provide neuroprotection from neonatal asphyxia. Ann Neurol 2005;58(2):182–93.

37. Martin JL, Ma D, Hossain M, et al. Asynchronous administration of xenon and hypothermia significantly reduces brain infarction in the neonatal rat. Br J Anaesth 2007;98(2):236–40.

38. Thoresen M, Hobbs CE, Wood T, et al. Cooling combined with immediate or delayed xenon inhalation provides equivalent long-term neuroprotection after neonatal hypoxia-ischemia. J Cereb Blood Flow Metab 2009;29(4):707–14.

39. Derwall M, Coburn M, Rex S, et al. Xenon: recent developments and future perspectives. Minerva Anestesiol 2009;75(1-2):37–45.

40. Dickinson R, Peterson BK, Banks P, et al. Competitive inhibition at the glycine site of the N-methyl-D-aspartate receptor by the anesthetics xenon and isoflurane: evidence from molecular modeling and electrophysiology. Anesthesiology 2007; 107(5):756–67.

41. Franks NP, Dickinson R, de Sousa SL, et al. How does xenon produce anaesthesia? Nature 1998;396(6709):324.

42. Weber NC, Toma O, Wolter JI, et al. Mechanisms of xenon- and isoflurane-induced preconditioning - a potential link to the cytoskeleton via the MAPKAPK-2/HSP27 pathway. Br J Pharmacol 2005;146(3):445–55.

43. Bantel C, Maze M, Trapp S. Noble gas xenon is a novel adenosine triphosphate-sensitive potassium channel opener. Anesthesiology 2010;112(3):623–30.

44. Gruss M, Bushell TJ, Bright DP, et al. Two-pore-domain K+ channels are a novel target for the anesthetic gases xenon, nitrous oxide, and cyclopropane. Mol Pharmacol 2004;65(2):443–52.

45. Coburn M, Maze M, Franks NP. The neuroprotective effects of xenon and helium in an in vitro model of traumatic brain injury. Crit Care Med 2008;36(2):588–95.
46. David HN, Leveille F, Chazalviel L, et al. Reduction of ischemic brain damage by nitrous oxide and xenon. J Cereb Blood Flow Metab 2003;23(10):1168–73.
47. Dingley J, Tooley J, Porter H, et al. Xenon provides short-term neuroprotection in neonatal rats when administered after hypoxia-ischemia. Stroke 2006;37(2):501–6.
48. Luo Y, Ma D, Ieong E, et al. Xenon and sevoflurane protect against brain injury in a neonatal asphyxia model. Anesthesiology 2008;109(5):782–9.
49. Ma D, Wilhelm S, Maze M, et al. Neuroprotective and neurotoxic properties of the 'inert' gas, xenon. Br J Anaesth 2002;89(5):739–46.
50. Schmidt M, Marx T, Gloggl E, et al. Xenon attenuates cerebral damage after ischemia in pigs. Anesthesiology 2005;102(5):929–36.
51. Fries M, Coburn M, Nolte KW, et al. Early administration of xenon or isoflurane may not improve functional outcome and cerebral alterations in a porcine model of cardiac arrest. Resuscitation 2009;80(5):584–90.
52. Chakkarapani E, Dingley J, Liu X, et al. Xenon enhances hypothermic neuroprotection in asphyxiated newborn pigs. Ann Neurol 2010;68(3):330–41.
53. Baumert JH, Hein M, Hecker KE, et al. Autonomic cardiac control with xenon anaesthesia in patients at cardiovascular risk. Br J Anaesth 2007;98(6):722–7.
54. Hartlage MA, Berendes E, Van Aken H, et al. Xenon improves recovery from myocardial stunning in chronically instrumented dogs. Anesth Analg 2004;99(3):655–64.
55. Preckel B, Mullenheim J, Moloschavij A, et al. Xenon administration during early reperfusion reduces infarct size after regional ischemia in the rabbit heart in vivo. Anesth Analg 2000;91(6):1327–32.
56. Baumert JH, Hecker KE, Hein M, et al. Haemodynamic effects of haemorrhage during xenon anaesthesia in pigs. Br J Anaesth 2005;94(6):727–32.
57. Francis RC, Philippi-Hohne C, Klein A, et al. Xenon/remifentanil anesthesia protects against adverse effects of losartan on hemodynamic challenges induced by anesthesia and acute blood loss. Shock 2010;34(6):628–35.
58. Wappler F, Rossaint R, Baumert J, et al. Multicenter randomized comparison of xenon and isoflurane on left ventricular function in patients undergoing elective surgery. Anesthesiology 2007;106(3):463–71.
59. Rossaint R, Reyle-Hahn M, Schulte Am Esch J, et al. Multicenter randomized comparison of the efficacy and safety of xenon and isoflurane in patients undergoing elective surgery. Anesthesiology 2003;98(1):6–13.
60. Laurent I, Monchi M, Chiche JD, et al. Reversible myocardial dysfunction in survivors of out-of-hospital cardiac arrest. J Am Coll Cardiol 2002;40(12):2110–6.
61. Tang W, Weil MH, Sun S, et al. Epinephrine increases the severity of postresuscitation myocardial dysfunction. Circulation 1995;92(10):3089–93.
62. Chen YS, Lin JW, Yu HY, et al. Cardiopulmonary resuscitation with assisted extracorporeal life-support versus conventional cardiopulmonary resuscitation in adults with in-hospital cardiac arrest: an observational study and propensity analysis. Lancet 2008;372(9638):554–61.
63. Kempski O. Pathologische neurophysiologie. In: Jantzen JP, Löffler W, editors. Neuroanästhesie. 1st edition. New York: Thieme; 2000. p. 91–4.
64. Nolan JP, Soar J, Zideman DA, et al. European Resuscitation Council Guidelines for Resuscitation 2010 Section 1. Executive summary. Resuscitation 2010;81(10):1219–76.

65. 2005 International Consensus on Cardiopulmonary Resuscitation and Emergency Cardiovascular Care Science with Treatment Recommendations. Part 3: defibrillation. Resuscitation 2005;67(2-3):203–11.
66. Delguercio LR, Feins NR, Cohn JD, et al. Comparison of blood flow during external and internal cardiac massage in man. Circulation 1965;31(Suppl 1):171–80.
67. Skorning M, Beckers SK, Brokmann J, et al. New visual feedback device improves performance of chest compressions by professionals in simulated cardiac arrest. Resuscitation 2010;81(1):53–8.
68. Derwall M, Francis RC, Kida K, et al. Administration of hydrogen sulfide via extracorporeal membrane lung ventilation in sheep with partial cardiopulmonary bypass perfusion: a proof of concept study on metabolic and vasomotor effects. Crit Care 2011;15(1):R51.
69. Keilegavlen H, Nordrehaug JE, Faerestrand S, et al. Treatment of cardiogenic shock with left ventricular assist device combined with cardiac resynchronization therapy: a case report. J Cardiothorac Surg 2010;5:54.
70. Manzo-Silberman S, Fichet J, Leprince P, et al. Cardiac arrest caused by coronary vasospasm treated with isosorbide dinitrate and left ventricular assistance. Resuscitation 2010;81(7):919–20.
71. Tuseth V, Pettersen RJ, Epstein A, et al. Percutaneous left ventricular assist device can prevent acute cerebral ischaemia during ventricular fibrillation. Resuscitation 2009;80(10):1197–203.
72. Tuseth V, Pettersen RJ, Grong K, et al. Randomised comparison of percutaneous left ventricular assist device with open-chest cardiac massage and with surgical assist device during ischaemic cardiac arrest. Resuscitation 2010;81(11):1566–70.
73. Tuseth V, Salem M, Pettersen R, et al. Percutaneous left ventricular assist in ischemic cardiac arrest. Crit Care Med 2009;37(4):1365–72.
74. Blackstone E, Morrison M, Roth MB. H2S induces a suspended animation-like state in mice. Science 2005;308(5721):518.
75. Blackstone E, Roth MB. Suspended animation-like state protects mice from lethal hypoxia. Shock 2007;27(4):370–2.
76. Roth MB, Nystul T. Buying time in suspended animation. Sci Am 2005;292(6):48–55.
77. Morrison ML, Blackwood JE, Lockett SL, et al. Surviving blood loss using hydrogen sulfide. J Trauma 2008;65(1):183–8.
78. Minamishima S, Bougaki M, Sips PY, et al. Hydrogen sulfide improves survival after cardiac arrest and cardiopulmonary resuscitation via a nitric oxide synthase 3-dependent mechanism in mice. Circulation 2009;120(10):888–96.
79. Derwall M, Westerkamp M, Lower C, et al. Hydrogen sulfide does not increase resuscitability in a porcine model of prolonged cardiac arrest. Shock 2010;34(2):190–5.
80. Olson KR, Dombkowski RA, Russell MJ, et al. Hydrogen sulfide as an oxygen sensor/transducer in vertebrate hypoxic vasoconstriction and hypoxic vasodilation. J Exp Biol 2006;209(Pt 20):4011–23.
81. Olson KR, Whitfield NL, Bearden SE, et al. Hypoxic pulmonary vasodilation: a paradigm shift with a hydrogen sulfide mechanism. Am J Physiol Regul Integr Comp Physiol 2010;298(1):R51–60.
82. Cai Z, Semenza GL. Phosphatidylinositol-3-kinase signaling is required for erythropoietin-mediated acute protection against myocardial ischemia/reperfusion injury. Circulation 2004;109(17):2050–3.
83. Fiordaliso F, Chimenti S, Staszewsky L, et al. A nonerythropoietic derivative of erythropoietin protects the myocardium from ischemia-reperfusion injury. Proc Natl Acad Sci U S A 2005;102(6):2046–51.

84. Cariou A, Claessens YE, Pene F, et al. Early high-dose erythropoietin therapy and hypothermia after out-of-hospital cardiac arrest: a matched control study. Resuscitation 2008;76(3):397–404.
85. Grmec S, Strnad M, Kupnik D, et al. Erythropoietin facilitates the return of spontaneous circulation and survival in victims of out-of-hospital cardiac arrest. Resuscitation 2009;80(6):631–7.

The Role of Emergency Coronary Intervention During and Following Cardiopulmonary Resuscitation

Sachin Kumar, MD, Elmer Murdock, MD,
Rajkumar K. Sugumaran, MD, Karl B. Kern, MD*

KEYWORDS

• Coronary intervention • Emergency medicine
• Cardiopulmonary resuscitation • Coronary angiography

The vast majority of patients with out-of-hospital cardiac arrest have underlying coronary artery disease. Autopsy studies have documented an 80% to 90% incidence of significant coronary disease in adults succumbing to sudden cardiac death.[1] Prospective studies of coronary angiography of those successfully resuscitated also show an incidence of coronary disease approaching 80%.[2] Acute coronary ischemia is a common trigger for out-of-hospital ventricular fibrillation cardiac arrest. Culprit lesions can be readily identified during coronary angiography immediately after resuscitation in 90% of those with ST elevation myocardial infarction (STEMI) and in 25% of those without STEMI.[3]

CARDIAC ARREST DURING CORONARY ANGIOGRAPHY AND PERCUTANEOUS CORONARY INTERVENTION

Coronary angiography remains the gold standard for diagnosing and treating coronary artery disease. Despite technological advances, cardiac catheterization carries a finite risk of morbidity and mortality. In a series of nearly 60,000 patients, the risk of all major complications from coronary angiography was less than 2%.[4] As with any medical procedure, death is the most dreaded complication, but the incidence is low, estimated to be 0.1%.[4] Although serious complications are rare, certain groups of patients are at higher risk. The stability of the patient before the

The authors have nothing to disclose.
Section of Cardiology, University of Arizona, Sarver Heart Center, 1501 North Campbell Avenue, Tucson, AZ 85724, USA
* Corresponding author.
E-mail address: kernk@email.arizona.edu

procedure significantly influences outcome, with the highest risk associated with patients who are moribund (tenfold increase) or in shock (sixfold increase).[5]

The incidence of death with percutaneous coronary intervention (PCI) is estimated at 1% (range, 0.5%–1.4%).[6] The incidence of cardiac arrest with PCI is more difficult to determine. Webb and colleagues[7] reported that in 4366 consecutive PCI patients, 57 had a cardiac arrest, for an overall incidence of 1.3%. Cardiac arrest was defined as cardiovascular collapse requiring cardiac resuscitation with or without defibrillation. Nearly half (47%) occurred during the PCI, whereas 53% occurred later that same day after leaving the cardiac catheterization suite. The majority of patients had an initial tachyarrhythmia, including ventricular fibrillation (36%) or ventricular tachycardia (28%). Bradyasystolic rhythms were less common but were seen, including bradycardia (24%), asystole (8%), and pulseless electrical activity (PEA) (2%). Predictors of cardiac arrest included emergency interventions, such as during an acute myocardial infarction, and cardiogenic shock. Percutaneous intervention of both the left anterior descending and right coronary artery were more commonly associated with cardiac arrest than was PCI of the left circumflex artery. Coronary angiography was repeated for the majority who had a cardiac arrest after leaving the PCI suite. A significant proportion had a major side branch occlusion (38%), persistent no-reflow (32%), or acute stent thrombosis (25%). Tamponade from distal wire perforation, undetected while in the catheterization laboratory, was found in one patient (4%). The vast majority of cardiac arrests (98%) occurred during an emergent PCI setting. Cardiac arrest was exceedingly rare during elective PCI cases, occurring in only 0.02% of such patients. Cardiac arrest associated with PCI is, however, not benign. The subsequent 24-hour mortality rate was 63%. Those most likely to die are the elderly and those in whom the cardiac arrest is associated with shock, no-reflow, side branch occlusion, or intraprocedural arrest. Although the overall incidence of cardiac arrest with PCI is low (1.3%), the majority of those who do arrest subsequently do poorly.

PREVENTION OF CARDIAC ARREST DURING PCI

President Eisenhower once said, "In preparing for battle, I have always found that plans are useless but planning is indispensable." Preinterventional planning is the single most important aspect of avoiding possible PCI complications including cardiac arrest. One needs to have a good understanding of the events that can lead to cardiac collapse and have an appropriate plan, including specific technology, should such a contingency be needed. Such technology should include functional defibrillators, temporary pacing equipment, circulatory support systems such as intraaortic balloon counterpulsation, and possibly the Impella (Abiomed) or extracorporeal membrane oxygenation systems.

TREATMENT STRATEGIES FOR CARDIAC ARREST DURING PCI

Several distinct scenarios can occur leading to cardiac arrest during PCI. Careful consideration of these circumstances before they occur can prepare one to recognize and appropriately treat each, despite the stress-filled environment when they do happen.

Hemodynamic Collapse

Sudden hypotension in the cardiac catheterization laboratory must be dealt with immediately if cardiac arrest is to be avoided. When troubleshooting abrupt hypotension, first make sure it is real. Check the position of the catheter through which the arterial pressure is measured. Pull back the guiding catheter to be sure it is not dampening the pressure measurement. Likewise, check for an open hemostatic Y-connector valve. If neither is the culprit, accept the pressure measurement as accurate and begin to consider possible causes. Acute hypotension can result from extensive vasodilation, including a profound vasovagal response, an anaphylactic reaction, medication overdose, severe bleeding, a tachyarrhythmia or bradyarrhythmia, perforation with cardiac tamponade, or extensive myocardial ischemia with subsequent left ventricular failure from either acute vessel closure or no-reflow. Emergent response depends on the cause but should include administration of fluids, raising the legs, and reversing any offending medications. Cardioversion or pacing may be needed for tachyarrhythmias or bradyarrhythmias, whereas emergent pericardiocentesis is almost always necessary for acute tamponade. Finally, if an acute epicardial vessel closure is discovered, reperfusion may be accomplished by either mechanical means, chemical thrombolysis, or a combination of the two. Successful treatment of microvascular no-flow requires intracoronary administration of chemical agents such as nicardipine, nitroprusside, or adenosine.

Ventricular Fibrillation Cardiac Arrest in the PCI Suite

Ventricular fibrillation cardiac arrest as a cause of acute hypotension should be readily recognized because electrocardiographic (ECG) monitoring is routine during coronary intervention. If defibrillation pads are already in place, immediate defibrillation can be performed. If not, the image intensifier should be moved from above the patient to allow access for placing pads or paddles in the standard left upper sternal and apical positions for optimal defibrillation. Sterile coverings must be removed to achieve pad-/paddle-to-skin contact. If paddles are used, conductive gel is needed for optimal contact and energy transfer. Defibrillation pads have such a gel in their adhesive. The 2010 cardiopulmonary resuscitation (CPR) guidelines recommend that a single maximal energy shock be delivered while no one else is touching the person.[8] If defibrillation fails, a second and even third shock should be considered in rapid sequence. If ventricular fibrillation persists, chest compressions should be started and the cause of the ventricular fibrillation sought. Several principles are important to remember when providing emergent circulatory support with chest compressions. First, chest compressions should be uninterrupted as nearly as possible. Ventricular fibrillation in the PCI suite should be immediately recognized, with chest compressions begun within a very short period of hemodynamic collapse. Therefore, ventilation will not be necessary for several minutes, and any attempt at endotracheal intubation or positive pressure ventilation should not be allowed to interrupt chest compressions. Forceful anterior-posterior chest compressions should be performed at 100 to 120 per minute. With the ability to measure aortic pressure via the indwelling catheters, strive for an aortic diastolic pressure (pressure during the relaxation portion of chest compressions) of at least 40 mmHg (the higher the better). This measure is the major determinant of coronary perfusion pressure during chest compressions. However, providing manual chest compressions for patients on the angiographic table is difficult at best and sometimes nearly impossible.

MECHANICAL CHEST COMPRESSION DEVICES IN THE CATHETERIZATION LABORATORY

Adequate circulatory support to both brain and heart is key for successful resuscitation from cardiac arrest, including cardiac arrest occurring in the catheterization suite. Mechanical chest compressors, developed as an alternative to manual compression, are ideal for providing compression-generated circulatory support in the

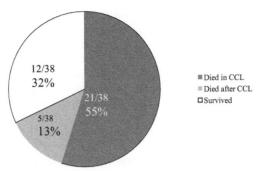

Fig. 1. Mechanical CPR for cardiac arrest in the catheterization suite, outcomes among 38 patients experiencing refractory cardiac arrest from acute coronary catastrophes occurring in the cardiac catheterization laboratory with the use of mechanical chest compressions. (*Data from* Wagner H, Terkelsen CJ, Friberg H, et al. Cardiac arrest in the catheterization laboratory: a 5-year experience of using mechanical chest compressions to facilitate PCI during prolonged resuscitation efforts. Resuscitation 2010;81:383–7.)

cardiac catheterization suite. When properly applied, mechanical chest compression devices have several theoretical advantages. They are not subject to fatigue, a common problem with manual chest compressions. They are consistent in the force and depth delivered, as determined by the operator. They can provide truly continuous chest compressions if not repeatedly interrupted and turned off. Such devices have one other unique advantage during PCI: they can provide chest compressions during fluoroscopy without irradiating the compressor's hands. Several reports of successful use of mechanical chest compression devices during arrest in the catheterization suite have been published in the last several years.[9–12] One of the devices that allows this is the Lund University Cardiopulmonary Assist System (LUCAS), a compressed air or battery-driven piston device providing mechanical chest compressions. This piston compression device incorporates a suction cup for active decompressions. The use of this device for performing prolonged chest compressions in cardiac arrest victims, either on their way to or in the cardiac catheterization suite, was first reported in 2005. Although the piston prohibits an anterior-posterior radiographic view, standard right anterior oblique, left anterior oblique, cranial, and caudal views (those views most commonly used in PCI) are all achievable.

The largest experience with LUCAS mechanical chest compressions for cardiac arrest in the catheterization laboratory was reported by Wagner and colleagues.[12] Over a period of 4 years (2004–2008), these investigators performed 6350 PCIs, of which 3058 were acute STEMI PCIs. Within this period, mechanical chest compressions were used in 43 patients with prolonged resuscitation efforts, typically requiring several minutes of manual chest compressions before beginning mechanical assistance. The age range was 31 to 86, with a mean age of 73. Forty-two of the 43 patients had coronary artery disease. Culprit coronary lesions were most often found in the left main (21%) or left anterior descending (60%) artery. Percutaneous coronary interventions were attempted in 36 of the 42 patients (86%) with coronary disease, of which 27 of 36 (75%) were considered technically successful. Causes of unsuccessful PCI included complex lesions, distal embolization, and no-reflow. The duration of mechanical chest compression averaged 28 minutes for the entire group and 17 minutes among survivors. (**Fig. 1**) is the outcomes flow chart for the 38 patients with an acute coronary catastrophe resulting in cardiac arrest who received mechanical chest compressions in the cardiac catheterization suite. Forty-five percent (17 of 38) were successfully resuscitated in the catheterization suite. Twelve survived to hospital discharge (32% of the whole group; 71% of those initially successfully resuscitated). A total of 11 of 38 patients (29%) were discharged with normal neurologic function (Cerebral Performance Category 1). Mechanical chest compressions allowed rescue interventions (PCI mostly, but also one case of successful pericardiocentesis) to be performed during ongoing resuscitation efforts. Almost certainly all of these patients would have died in the catheterization laboratory but for this technology. The investigators note that coronary angiography is always feasible with ongoing mechanical compressions, whereas the actual stent placement can be done with precision by temporarily pausing the mechanical compressions to allow exact positioning before deployment. This experience once again showed that most often such cases are associated with STEMIs. Although infrequent, only 33 out of 3058 patients (1.1%) with STEMI had refractory cardiac arrest in the catheterization suite.

Although mechanical chest compressions have been lifesaving for some arresting in the cardiac catheterization laboratory, particularly those who have a remediable cause of their arrest, compressions have not generally worked well for those with refractory cardiac arrest occurring outside of the catheterization suite. This approach was attempted in 13 patients in a report by Larsen and colleagues.[11] These investigators showed that mechanical chest compressions with LUCAS could maintain adequate organ perfusion while continuing to pursue PCI. In their series, the mean duration of mechanical compressions was 105±60 minutes (range, 45–240), and the mean systolic and diastolic blood pressures obtained were 81±23 and 34±21 mmHg, respectively. Angiography, and eventually PCI, were possible in all cases during ongoing automatic chest compression. Three patients (23%) survived the catheterization laboratory procedure, but no patient survived to hospital discharge. This result is another example that timely therapy remains key to long-term, successful neurologically-intact survival.[13]

Another device is the AutoPulse, an automated portable battery-powered CPR device manufactured by ZOLL Medical Corporation. This mechanical chest compression device is composed of a constricting band and backboard. The device has been used in refractory cardiac arrest in the cardiac catheterization laboratory successfully but is limited to cranial and caudal views because of the radiopaque circuitry in the backboard.

Emergency percutaneous cardiopulmonary bypass has been used in refractory cardiac arrest occurring in the catheterization laboratory. Excellent systemic perfusion support can be accomplished with such technology, allowing definitive therapy to be attempted with either PCI or coronary artery bypass graft for those with unresponsive cardiac arrest. Several small series of such patients were reported in the 1990s, generally with good survival rates.[14–17] Of the 26 patients reported in the literature, 18 (69%) survived to hospital discharge.

Percutaneous left ventricular assist devices now exist and have found favor for enhanced hemodynamic support during high-risk PCI.[18] However, their role in actual cardiac arrest is only now beginning to be evaluated. Tuseth and colleagues[19] in Norway reported that during 15 minutes of untreated ventricular fibrillation, the Impella 2.5 pump was able to provide nearly 70% of prearrest cerebral and myocardial flows. Intensive volume administration (1.5 mL/kg/min) helped maintain similar flows for 30 minutes, but no attempt at defibrillation or resuscitation was performed, so no outcome data are available. The role of such a pump inserted percutaneously during cardiac arrest in the catheterization laboratory is currently only speculative.

CORONARY ANGIOGRAPHY AFTER RESUSCITATION FROM CARDIAC ARREST

For a long time it was commonly thought that survival from out-of-hospital cardiac arrest was a reflection of timely interventions performed in the prehospital setting. It is now recognized that successful resuscitation does not end at the return of spontaneous circulation (ROSC) and that much more can be done to achieve long-term survival with favorable neurologic function. Extensive experimental work along with astute clinical observations in the past 2 decades have provided significant insights into the pathophysiology of cardiac arrest.[20,21] Cardiac arrest causes global ischemia affecting multiple organ systems. Restoration of spontaneous circulation sets the milieu for reperfusion injury to the same organs and tissues.[22] Cardiac stunning with resultant myocardial dysfunction along with neurologic injury are the main predictors of outcome during the postarrest period. A number of postresuscitation strategies have been followed in an attempt to improve outcomes. The two most consistently shown to be of promise in improving meaningful long-term neurologic survival are (a) induction of mild therapeutic hypothermia and (b) early coronary angiography and intervention.

The usefulness of hypothermia in cardiac arrest patients is not a new discovery. The beneficial effects of hypothermia after cold water drowning have long been known. Moderate and severe hypothermia after resuscitation was attempted in the early 1960s with inconclusive results because of a high incidence of complications. Two randomized clinical trials in the last decade found that mild hypothermia (32–34°C) improved both survival and neurologic function of those survivors among comatose adult patients resuscitated from out-of-hospital ventricular fibrillation.[23,24] These studies did not use concurrent urgent revascularization. Based on the preclinical experiments, it would seem logical to use hypothermia in the setting of a cardiac arrest associated with a myocardial infarction because therapeutic hypothermia has been shown to reduce infarct size.[25] However, there were initial concerns over combining therapeutic hypothermia and early revascularization strategy in clinical practice. Hypothermia has been associated with platelet dysfunction, activation of fibrinolysis cascade, coagulation abnormalities, electrolyte and intravascular volume shifts, and arrhythmias. These associations seem to be counterintuitive to the concept of safely performing coronary intervention, which requires use of anticoagulants and antiplatelet therapies, thus increasing the risk of bleeding and hence mortality associated with this procedure.

There is now abundant clinical evidence that hypothermia combined with early coronary angiography postresuscitation is both safe and efficacious. Numerous observational clinical reports have demonstrated that not only is this strategy safe, but it also provides meaningful survival benefit. Data from survivors of cardiac arrest in Oslo and Melbourne highlighted the importance of using a standardized protocol, which includes routine use of therapeutic hypothermia along with early angiography/ intervention resulting in doubling of overall and neurologic survival in their patient populations.[26,27] Various studies have looked at the impact of bleeding and other complications and have proposed the safety and feasibility of this combined approach.[27,28] The group from Oslo published an update of their previous experience. In the 5 years following their first report, postresuscitation hypothermia and early coronary intervention produced the same good results, with 56% overall survival rate. Additionally, 93% of all survivors had favorable neurologic function, suggesting that

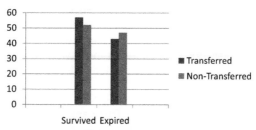

Fig. 2. Survival after cardiac arrest according to transfer status. No differences in outcomes were found between those with cardiac arrests resuscitated locally and those arresting and resuscitated in outlying referral areas requiring transfer to the central referral center. (*Data from* Mooney MR, Unger BT, Boland LL, et al. Therapeutic hypothermia after out-of-hospital cardiac arrest: evaluation of a regional system to increase access to cooling. Circulation 2011;124(2):206–14.)

the improvements in survival are not at the expense of patient independence or cognitive function.

Stub and Australian colleagues[27] reported their single-center experience in combining therapeutic hypothermia with early coronary angiography and intervention in 125 patients.[27] They found that the combination of hypothermia and early coronary intervention resulted in significantly better survival to discharge compared with their historical control rates (64% vs 39%; $P = .01$) and resulted in more intact neurologic function among survivors (88% vs 76%; $P<.01$).

Recent results from the Cool It strategy by Mooney and colleagues[29] echoed the findings from several other similar single-center or multicenter registries. Cool It is an initiative implemented by the Minneapolis Heart Institute with the aim to improve neurologic outcome by ensuring that all the survivors of out-of-hospital cardiac arrest receive therapeutic hypothermia through a regionalized systems approach that includes early angiography in patients with ST elevation.[9] They reported on 140 out-of-hospital cardiac arrest patients, three-quarters (n = 107) of whom were transferred to the therapeutic hypothermia receiving center from the referring network hospitals. Patients with evidence of STEMI (n = 68) postresuscitation received emergent coronary angiography and intervention while being cooled. Overall survival to hospital discharge was 56%, with 92% of survivors having good neurologic function. No differences in outcomes were noted between transferred and nontransferred patients (**Fig. 2**). This result is an example of how an established regional STEMI system of care can be further developed into a postresuscitation care network, extending lifesaving therapeutic hypothermia to many additional cardiac arrest victims.

Use of therapeutic hypothermia is currently recommended in patients who remain comatose post–cardiac arrest and present with an initial shockable rhythm; however, there is considerable disagreement regarding its potential role in victims with asystole/PEA. The original American Heart Association (AHA)/International Liaison Committee on Resuscitation (ILCOR) guidelines did not directly endorse the use of therapeutic hypothermia in this group but stated that it might be useful and could be considered for such therapy.[30] Although the mortality in patients with asystole/PEA remains high, recent experience from the Hypothermia Registry Network suggests that if such patients are cooled and survive, they have rates of successful neurologic recovery comparable with cooled survivors of ventricular fibrillation cardiac arrest.[31] It seems that if patients survive the insult of cardiac arrest and are discharged from the hospital, they have a very good chance of successful neurologic recovery. Nearly 90% of resuscitated victims of out-of-hospital ventricular fibrillation who survive to discharge are neurologically intact. These recent data from Mooney[29] and the Hypothermia Registry Network[31] suggest that those with non–ventricular fibrillation cardiac arrest should be cooled postresuscitation to achieve the best long-term outcomes.

Autopsy studies from cardiac arrest victims have revealed a high prevalence of occlusive coronary disease in this subset.[1] There are also clinical data on incidence of significant coronary artery disease in cardiac arrest patients. Spaulding and colleagues[2] in 1997 proposed the idea of performing coronary angiography in patients who presented to the hospital after successful resuscitation from cardiac arrest with no other obvious noncardiac cause of arrest. Their hypothesis was based on the fact that a large proportion of these patients have an underlying acute ischemic milieu, and urgent coronary intervention could make a difference. Eighty-four patients meeting the entry criteria were enrolled in the study to undergo coronary angiography. Several valuable clinical observations were made from this landmark study. The investigators found that on angiography, nearly two-thirds of victims had evidence of significant coronary artery disease (>70% stenosis) with complete occlusion evident in half of the patients. Successful coronary intervention was shown to be an independent predictor of survival in multivariate analysis.

Another important observation from the study was the lack of predictability of the clinical and ECG variables to consistently diagnose significant coronary artery disease in this population. This result is very different from routine practice in the general population, in which ischemic ECG findings drive clinical practice guidelines. The Spaulding study introduced the concept of performing coronary angiography and interventions in cardiac arrest patients, not based solely on the ECG findings, and demonstrated improvement in outcome among those so treated.[2]

Because the demonstration by Spaulding that emergent coronary angiography could be safely performed in the post–cardiac arrest patient, various observational studies supporting this approach have been published. It has been observed by various investigators that when primary angioplasty is performed in patients who have a post–cardiac arrest perfusing rhythm and ST elevation on the electrocardiogram, the overwhelming majority (more than 75% of these patients) have acute coronary occlusion and the remaining have high-grade coronary stenosis.[27,28,32–34] Several observational studies have demonstrated that patients who are alert at presentation to the hospital after being resuscitated in the field have a better chance of successful neurologic outcome when compared with patients who are comatose.[32,33] However, it is well-known that ability to predict recovery based on the level of consciousness at presentation is poor. These patients, despite a more guarded prognosis than the alert patients, still have a reasonable chance for good outcomes and should be offered the same treatment. Use of therapeutic hypothermia in patients remaining comatose after resuscitation has resulted in dramatic improvement in neurologic survival.

From the growing body of evidence in post–cardiac arrest patients, it is now recognized that there are certain variables that predict chances of successful neurologic recovery once these patients are resuscitated. Shorter times to initiation of bystander CPR and ROSC after the cardiac arrest, younger age, neurologic status at the time of in-hospital presentation (alert vs comatose), ventricular fibrillation as the presenting rhythm, presence of STEMI on the presenting electrocardiogram, and absence of diabetes are predictors of better outcome at 1 and 6 months.[1,26,32] Although such features are favorable, their absence should not prevent the treatment of patients with a less favorable presentation.

In certain parts of the world primary angioplasty is not immediately available, and in such instances successful use of thrombolytics has been proposed as an alternative in an effort to improve neurologic recovery.[35] However, where primary angioplasty is available, it remains the approach of choice. The AHA and ILCOR groups incorporated in their new 2010 International Consensus on Cardiopulmonary Resuscitation and Emergency Cardiovascular Care Science With Treatment Recommendations statements supporting the use of coronary angiography and PCI after successful resuscitation from out-of-hospital cardiac arrest.[36] They note the following:

> In OHCA (out-of-hospital cardiac arrest) patients with STEMI or new LBBB (left bundle branch block) on ECG following ROSC, early angiography and PPCI (primary PCI) should be considered. It is reasonable to perform early angiography and PPCI in selected patients despite the absence of ST-segment elevation on the ECG or prior clinical findings, such as chest pain, if coronary ischemia is considered the likely cause on clinical grounds. Out-of-hospital cardiac arrest patients are often initially comatose but this should not be a contraindication to consider immediate angiography and PCI. It may be reasonable to include cardiac catheterization in a standardized post–cardiac-arrest protocol as part of an overall strategy to improve neurologically intact survival in this patient group. Therapeutic hypothermia is recommended in combination with primary PCI, and should be started as early as possible, preferably before initiation of PCI.

The AHA likewise suggested in their 2010 Guidelines for Cardiopulmonary Resuscitation and Emergency Cardiovascular Care that PCI following ROSC after cardiac arrest is a Class I, "Level of Evidence" B class (LOE B) recommendation for patients with ventricular fibrillation cardiac arrest in the setting of ST elevation or new LBBB.[37,38] They note, "Angiography and/or PCI need not preclude or delay other therapeutic strategies including therapeutic hypothermia (Class IIa, LOE B)."

But is the same approach with emergent coronary angiography and therapeutic hypothermia effective for those who present with ventricular fibrillation arrest but do not have evidence of ST elevation? What of those with other ECG patterns such as ST depression, conduction abnormalities, and nonspecific ST-T changes? It has been well-accepted that these patients should receive therapeutic hypothermia if they remain comatose after resuscitation, but their need for concurrent urgent coronary angiography is not yet well-defined. One aspect of this dilemma as noted by Spaulding and colleagues[2] is the poor sensitivity of ECG in identifying underlying ischemic triggers in cardiac arrest patients. This problem leads to the question, are some of these non-ST elevation cardiac arrest patients being denied optimal therapy? Data gathered from observations from the French PROCAT (Parisian Region Out-of-Hospital Cardiac Arrest) Registry, which represents the largest cohort of patients with post–cardiac arrest and angiographic data yet published, reveal that when these patients undergo routine coronary angiography, an acute culprit lesion is identified in half of them.[39] PROCAT investigators and others researchers have shown that successful revascularization is associated with improved survival and is an independent predictor regardless of the ECG pattern (**Fig. 3**).[3,39,40] This area still remains open to debate, but the AHA notes in its 2010 Guidelines for Cardiopulmonary Resuscitation and Emergency Cardiovascular Care, "Primary PCI also appears applicable in the setting of NSTEMI (non-STEMI) subjects in whom emergent revascularization may result in hemodynamic and electric stability. PPCI after ROSC

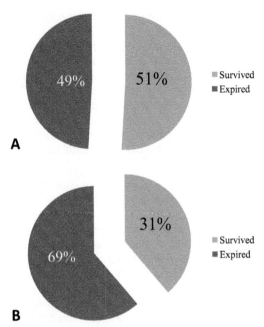

Fig. 3. Survival depends on successful PCI. Marked differences in outcome were noted between those with successful percutaneous coronary intervention (*A*) and those with unsuccessful or no attempt at percutaneous coronary intervention (*B*). (*Data from* Dumas F, Cariou A, Manzo-Silberman S, et al. Immediate percutaneous coronary intervention is associated with better survival after out-of-hospital cardiac arrest: insights from the PROCAT (Parisian Region Out of hospital Cardiac ArresT) registry. Circ Cardiovasc Interv 2010;3(3):200–7.)

in subjects with arrest of presumed ischemic cardiac etiology may be reasonable, even in the absence of a clearly defined STEMI (Class IIb, LOE B)."[37]

FINDING THE RIGHT PATIENT FOR POST CARDIAC ARREST EMERGENT CORONARY ANGIOGRAPHY

After a decade of experience, certain prognostic features suggest who is likely to benefit from emergency cardiac catheterization after cardiac arrest. This population includes younger patients, those with ventricular fibrillation cardiac arrest, those with short periods from cardiac arrest to ROSC, those with ST elevation postarrest, and those who are awake after resuscitation. The contrary features are associated with less chance of good outcomes but nonetheless can still incrementally benefit from aggressive postresuscitation care. Sideris and colleagues[41] in France recently suggested that although the lack of ST elevation is not evidence of a noncardiac cause of arrest, the combined criteria of ST segment elevation and/or depression and/or a wide QRS bundle branch pattern was very sensitive in identifying cardiac cause in out-of-hospital arrest victims. The investigators found that such criteria provided a sensitivity and negative predictive value for detecting acute myocardial infarction postarrest of 100%. However, the authors' Arizona experience[42] and that of others[3,38] differ in that the authors found that a completely normal postarrest ECG did not completely rule out acute coronary occlusions or unstable thrombotic lesions.

Box 1
Suggested elements for a regional cardiac resuscitation center

Cooperative relationship with the local EMS services

Aligned with regional STEMI centers

External certification, not self-designation

Capable of providing therapeutic hypothermia

Capable of primary PCI 24/7

Minimum of 40 postresuscitation patients per year

Capable of treating those who rearrest, including mechanical options

Capable of EP testing and ICD implantation

Provide public CPR training

Provide professional CPR training

Defer assessment of prognosis for 72 hours postcooling

Multidisciplinary approach to cardiac arrest victims including EMS, emergency medicine, Cardiology, neurology, and critical care specialists.

Abbreviations: EP, electrophysiology; ICD, implantable cardioverter defibrillator.

Data from Nichols G, Aufderheide TP, Eigel B, et al. Regional systems of care for out-of-hospital cardiac arrest. Circulation 2010;121:709–29.

CARDIAC ARREST CENTERS: PROVIDING CORONARY ANGIOGRAPHY AND PCI TO THE POSTRESUSCITATED

In order to provide optimal care including mild therapeutic hypothermia and early coronary angiography/PCI to those resuscitated from out-of-hospital cardiac arrest, regionalized cardiac arrest centers have been proposed. Designated centers for specialized and dedicated postresuscitation care have been attractive because of the wide variation in survival rates depending on geographic location in both Europe[43] and the United States.[44,45] The AHA has issued a policy statement supporting such centers and the preliminary recommended elements of such systems, although the actual setup and operation of them remains somewhat vague and nonstandardized.[46] **Box 1** contains the specific recommendations made in this policy statement.

The Minneapolis Heart Institute has been a leader in establishing a regional system to extend optimal post–cardiac arrest care to more patients. In 2006, they began an initiative aimed at improving survival and neurologic recovery after cardiac arrest by affording regional and timely access to postresuscitation care using their well-established regional STEMI network.[47] Mooney and colleagues[29] used their long-standing relationships with a network of 33 hospitals in Minnesota and northern Wisconsin for transfer of patients needing emergent cardiovascular care (STEMI) in order to create a unique post–cardiac arrest treatment regional network. A new protocol for treatment and transfer of resuscitated cardiac arrest patients was implemented within this regional network. Patients were eligible if they were resuscitated but remained comatose and the time from collapse to ROSC was less than 60 minutes. Postarrest patients were eligible regardless of age, initial rhythm, postarrest ECG findings (STEMI or not), or hemodynamic stability. Prehospital cooling was recommended with ice, particularly among those being transferred. Upon arrival at

---

Box 2
Primary criteria for an Arizona cardiac arrest center

Agreement to provide appropriate postresuscitation care to all such victims

Agreement to collect and submit data to the state EMS office

Capability to provide therapeutic hypothermia 24/7

Capability to provide primary PCI 24/7

Commitment to evidence-based prognostication guidelines

Commitment to organ procurement

Agreement to public outreach to teach bystander CPR in their communities

Submission of at least 6 months of local baseline out-of-hospital cardiac arrest outcomes data

---

the receiving hospital, therapeutic hypothermia was continued with a mechanical surface-cooling device. Any patient with STEMI underwent emergent coronary angiography for potential PCI while being simultaneously cooled. Finally, systematic neurologic evaluation and treatment were also part of the Cool It program. Among the first 140 patients treated within the Cool It program, 56% survived to discharge, and 92% of all survivors had a favorable neurologic outcome.[29]

Arizona was first in the United States to implement a statewide program for post–cardiac arrest care. Beginning in 2007 under the direction of the Governor's office and through the authority of the state emergency medical services (EMS) director, voluntary agreement was sought with individual medical centers throughout the state to provide continuous access (24 hours a day, 7 days a week) for postresuscitated patients to (1) therapeutic hypothermia and (2) early coronary angiography and PCI.[48] Initially enthusiasm was low, but after an observational study found that transfer time was not related to survival, allowing EMS to bypass hospitals not prepared to provide full postresuscitation care, many hospitals readily applied so as not to be denied such patients.[49] The primary criteria for becoming a cardiac arrest center in Arizona are shown in **Box 2**. The overall goal was to provide a majority of out-of-hospital cardiac arrest victims in Arizona with standardized guide-based post–cardiac arrest care. Designations of cardiac arrest centers were made upon agreement with the stated conditions by the state EMS director's office. There was no fee for such a designation. Early experience seems to be positive with improvement in use of proven post–cardiac arrest therapies, and more important, improved outcomes among those suffering out-of-hospital cardiac arrest.

SUMMARY

Cardiac arrest during coronary angiography is rare, occurring in less than 0.1%. This incidence increases to 1.3% during PCIs. If, however, cardiac arrest does occur during cardiac catheterization and fails to respond quickly to standard resuscitation efforts, mechanical chest compression devices can be lifesaving. Such devices allow continued efforts at corrective action, generally emergency PCI during chest compressions, with approximately one-third of such patients surviving long-term with good neurologic function. Coronary angiography after successful resuscitation should be done whenever a cardiac cause for the arrest is suspected. Combining early coronary angiography and mild therapeutic hypothermia is the best strategy for improving long-term neurologically intact survival in those successfully resuscitated.

Cardiac arrest centers seem to be the best option for providing more cardiac arrest victims with aggressive postresuscitation care.

REFERENCES

1. Davies MJ, Thomas A. Thrombosis and acute coronary artery lesions in sudden cardiac ischemic death. N Engl J Med 1984;310:1137–40.
2. Spaulding CM, Joly LM, Rosenberg A, et al. Immediate coronary angiography in survivors of out-of-hospital cardiac arrest. N Engl J Med 1997;336(23):1629–33.
3. Radsel P, Knafelj R, Kocjancic S, et al. Angiographic characteristics of coronary disease and postresuscitation electrocardiograms in patients with aborted cardiac arrest outside a hospital. Am J Cardiol 2011;108:634–8.
4. Noto TJ Jr, Johnson LW, Krone R, et al. Cardiac catheterization 1990: a report of the Registry of the Society for Cardiac Angiography and Interventions (SCA&I). Cathet Cardiovasc Diagn 1991;24:75–83.
5. Laskey W, Boyle J, Johnson LW. Multivariable model for prediction of risk of significant complication during diagnostic cardiac catheterization: the Registry Committee of the Society for Cardiac Angiography and Interventions. Cathet Cardiovasc Diagn 1993; 30:185–90.
6. Smith SC, Dove JT, Jacobs AK, et al. ACC/AHA guidelines for percutaneous coronary intervention (revision of the 1993 guidelines). Circulation 2001;103:3019–41.
7. Webb JG, Solankhi NK, Chugh SK, et al. Incidence, correlates, and outcomes of cardiac arrest associated with percutaneous coronary intervention. Am J Cardiol 2002;90:1252–4
8. Link M, Atkins DL, Passman RS, et al. Part 6: electrical therapies: automatic external defibrillators, defibrillation, cardioversion, and pacing: 2010 American Heart Association guidelines for cardiopulmonary resuscitation and emergency cardiovascular care. Circulation 2010;122:(Suppl 3):S706–19.
9. Grogaard HK, Wik L, Eriksen M, et al. Continuous mechanical chest compressions during cardiac arrest to facilitate restoration of coronary circulation with percutaneous coronary intervention. J Am Coll Cardiol 2007;50:1093–109.
10. Agostoni P, Cornelis K, Vermeersch P. Successful percutaneous treatment of an intraprocedural left main stent thrombosis with the support of an automatic mechanical chest compression device. Int J Cardiol 2008;124:e19–21.
11. Larsen AI, Hjørnevik AS, Ellingsen CL, et al, Cardiac arrest with continuous mechanical chest compression during percutaneous coronary intervention. A report on the use of the LUCAS device. Resuscitation 2007;75:454–9.
12. Wagner H, Terkelsen CJ, Friberg H, et al. Cardiac arrest in the catheterization laboratory: a 5-year experience of using mechanical chest compressions to facilitate PCI during prolonged resuscitation efforts. Resuscitation 2010;81:383–7.
13. Kern KB, Sanders AB, Badylak SF, et al. The limitations of open chest cardiac massage after prolonged untreated cardiac arrest in dogs. Ann Emerg Med 1991;20: 761–7.
14. Shawl FA, Domanski MJ, Wish MH, et al. Emergency cardiopulmonary bypass support in patients with cardiac arrest in the catheterization laboratory. Cathet Cardiovasc Diagn 1990;19:8–12.
15. Overlie PA. Emergent use of portable cardiopulmonary bypass. Cathet Cardiovasc Diagn 1990;20:27–31.
16. Mooney MR, Arom KV, Joyce LD, et al. Emergency cardiopulmonary bypass support in patients with cardiac arrest. J Thorac Cardiovasc Surg 1991;101:450–4.

17. Redle J, King B, Lemoe G, et al. Utility of rapid percutaneous cardiopulmonary bypass for refractory hemodynamic collapse in the cardiac catheterization laboratory. Am J Cardiol 1994;73:899–900.
18. Sjauw K, Konorza T, Erbel R, et al. Supported high risk percutaneous coronary intervention with the Impella 2.5 device. J Am Coll Cardiol 2009;54:2430–4.
19. Tuseth V, Salem M, Pettersen R, et al. Percutaneous left ventricular assist in ischemic cardiac arrest. Crit Care Med 2009;37:365–72.
20. Laver S, Farrow C, Turner D, et al. Mode of death after admission to an intensive care unit following cardiac arrest. Intensive Care Med 2004;30:2126–8.
21. Kern KB. Postresuscitation myocardial dysfunction. Cardiol Clin 2002;20:89–101.
22. Nolan JP, Neumar RW, Adrie C, et al. Post-cardiac arrest syndrome: epidemiology, pathophysiology, treatment, and prognostication: a scientific statement from the International Liaison Committee on Resuscitation; the American Heart Association Emergency Cardiovascular Care Committee; the Council on Cardiovascular Surgery and Anesthesia; the Council on Cardiopulmonary, Perioperative, and Critical Care; the Council on Clinical Cardiology; the Council on Stroke (Part II). Int Emerg Nurs 2010;18(1):8–28.
23. Hypothermia after Cardiac Arrest Study Group. Mild therapeutic hypothermia to improve the neurologic outcome after cardiac arrest. N Engl J Med 2002;346(8): 549–56.
24. Bernard SA, Gray TW, Buist MD, et al. Treatment of comatose survivors of out-of-hospital cardiac arrest with induced hypothermia. N Engl J Med 2002;346(8):557–63.
25. Dae MA, Gao DW, Sessler DI, et al. Effect of endovascular cooling on myocardial temperature, infarct size, and cardiac output in human-sized pigs. Am J Physiol Heart Circ Physiol 2002;282:H1584–91.
26. Tømte O, Andersen GØ, Jacobsen D, et al. Strong and weak aspects of an established post-resuscitation treatment protocol-A five-year observational study. Resuscitation 2011;82(9):1186–93.
27. Stub D, Hengel C, Chan W, et al. Usefulness of cooling and coronary catheterization to improve survival in out-of-hospital cardiac arrest. Am J Cardiol 2011;107(4):522–7.
28. Schefold JC, Storm C, Joerres A, et al. Mild therapeutic hypothermia after cardiac arrest and the risk of bleeding in patients with acute myocardial infarction. Int J Cardiol.2009;132(3):387–91.
29. Mooney MR, Unger BT, Boland LL, et al. Therapeutic hypothermia after out-of-hospital cardiac arrest: evaluation of a regional system to increase access to cooling. Circulation 2011;124(2):206–14.
30. Nolan JP, Morley PT, Van den Hoek TL, et al. Therapeutic hypothermia after cardiac arrest: an advisory statement by the advanced life support task force of the International Liaison Committee on Resuscitation. Resuscitation 2003;57:231–5.
31. Nielsen N, Hovdenes J, Nilsson F, et al; for the Hypothermia Network. Outcome, timing and adverse events in therapeutic hypothermia after out-of-hospital cardiac arrest. Acta Anaesthesiol Scand 2009;53:926–34.
32. Garot P, Lefevre T, Eltchaninoff H, et al. Six-month outcome of emergency percutaneous coronary intervention in resuscitated patients after cardiac arrest complicating ST-elevation myocardial infarction. Circulation 2007;115(11):1354–62.
33. Hosmane VR, Mustafa NG, Reddy VK, et al. Survival and neurologic recovery in patients with ST-segment elevation myocardial infarction resuscitated from cardiac arrest. J Am Coll Cardiol 2009;53(5):409–15.
34. Gorjup V, Radsel P, Kocjancic ST, et al. Acute ST-elevation myocardial infarction after successful cardiopulmonary resuscitation. Resuscitation 2007;72(3):379–85.

35. Richling N, Herkner H, Holzer M, et al. Thrombolytic therapy vs primary percutaneous intervention after ventricular fibrillation cardiac arrest due to acute ST-segment elevation myocardial infarction and its effect on outcome. Am J Emerg Med. 2007; 25(5):545–50.

36. O'Connor RE, Bossaert L, Arntz H-R, et al. Part 9: acute coronary syndromes: 2010 International Consensus on Cardiopulmonary Resuscitation and Emergency Cardio-vascular Care Science with Treatment Recommendations. Circulation 2010;122(Suppl 2): S422–65.

37. O'Connor RE, Brady W, Brooks SC, et al. Part 10: acute coronary syndromes: 2010 AHA Guidelines for Cardiopulmonary Resuscitation and Emergency Cardiovascular Care. Circulation 2010;122(Suppl 3):S787–817.

38. Sayre M, O'Connor RE, Atkins D, et al. Part 2: evidence evaluation and management of potential or preceived conflict of interest: 2010 American Heart Association Guidelines for Cardiopulmonary Resuscitation and Emergency Cardiovascular Care. Circulation 2010;122(Suppl 3):S657–64.

39. Dumas F, Cariou A, Manzo-Silberman S, et al. Immediate percutaneous coronary intervention is associated with better survival after out-of-hospital cardiac arrest: insights from the PROCAT (Parisian Region Out of hospital Cardiac ArresT) registry. Circ Cardiovasc Interv 2010;3(3):200–7.

40. Cronier P, Vignon P, Bouferrache K, et al. Impact of routine percutaneous coronary intervention after out-of-hospital cardiac arrest due to ventricular fibrillation. Crit Care 2011;15(3):R122.

41. Sideris G, Voicu S, Dillinger J-G, et al. Value of post-resuscitation electrocardiogram in the diagnosis of acute myocardial infarction in out-of-hospital cardiac arrest patients. Resuscitation 2011;82:1148–53.

42. Kern KB, Rahman O. Emergent percutaneous coronary intervention for resuscitated victims of out-of-hospital cardiac arrest. Catheter Cardiovasc Interv 2010;75:616–24.

43. Herlitz J, Engdahl J, Svensson L, et al. Major differences in 1-month survival between hospitals in Sweden among initial survivors of out-of-hospital cardiac arrest. Resus-citation 2006;70:404–9.

44. Nichol G, Thomas E, Callaway CW, et al. Regional variation in out-of-hospital cardiac arrest incidence and outcome. JAMA 2008;300:1423–31.

45. Sanders AB, Kern KB. Surviving cardiac arrest: location, location, location. JAMA 2008;300:1462–3.

46. Nichols G, Aufderheide TP, Eigel B, et al. Regional systems of care for out-of-hospital cardiac arrest. Circulation 2010;121:709–29.

47. Henry TD, Sharkey SW, Burke N, et al. A regional system to provide timely access to percutaneous coronary intervention for ST-elevation myocardial infarction. Circulation 2007;116:721–8

48. Bobrow BJ, Kern KB. Regionalization of postcardiac arrest care. Curr Opin Crit Care 2009;15:221–7.

49. Spaite DW, Bobrow BJ, Vadeboncoeur TF, et al. The impact of prehospital transport interval on survival in out-of-hospital cardiac arrest: implications for regionalization of post-resuscitation care. Resuscitation 2008;79:61–6.

BONUS ARTICLE:
Risk Stratification for
Acute Pulmonary Embolism

Jason A. Stamm, MD

Edited by Kenneth E. Wood, DO

Risk Stratification for Acute Pulmonary Embolism

Jason A. Stamm, MD

KEYWORDS

• Pulmonary embolism • Prognosis • Risk • Outcomes

Pulmonary embolism (PE) is a commonly encountered condition in the medical and surgical intensive care unit. Whereas overall mortality in those with PE is 5% to 15% in the first few months after diagnosis due to a combination of underlying medical conditions, recurrent venous thromboembolism and right heart failure, outcomes after acute PE vary substantially across subgroups.[1–5] Patients who present with shock suffer from an approximate 25% to 50% short-term mortality rate, whereas those with preserved blood pressure at presentation experience only a 2% to 5% risk of death.[4–7] Despite this understanding of the spectrum of prognoses in those with acute PE, there remains much uncertainty in how best to align the risk of adverse outcome in acute PE with the appropriate intensity of therapeutic intervention. Apart from those who present in shock and immediately declare their prognosis, which patients with acute PE are at low risk of adverse outcomes and do not require a higher level of care? Which patients are at an elevated risk of clinical deterioration and should be treated in the intensive care unit and perhaps considered for thrombolytic therapy?

An understanding of the pathophysiology of acute PE is essential to risk stratification. Outcome in acute PE is dependent on the presence of preexisting comorbidities and the extent of hemodynamic compromise. Specifically, in the context of any underlying cardiopulmonary disease, the ability of the right ventricle (RV) to compensate for an increase in pulmonary vascular resistance is the major determinant of survival. The resistance to flow from the RV in acute PE is multifactorial and includes not only mechanical obstruction of the proximal pulmonary arteries by acute and/or recurrent thrombus but also the actions of humoral factors that are released from the clot, resulting in pulmonary vasoconstriction.[8,9] In addition, the hypoxemia that results from impaired ventilation/perfusion matching further increases pulmonary vascular resistance. Acutely, the RV can only compensate for a mean pulmonary artery pressure of approximately 40 mmHg, whereas much higher pulmonary pressures are tolerated if pulmonary hypertension (PH) occurs more gradually.[10,11] With

The author has nothing to disclose.

Division of Pulmonary and Critical Care Medicine, Mail Code 01-11, Geisinger Medical Center, 100 North Academy Avenue, Danville, PA 17822, USA

E-mail address: jastamm@geisinger.edu

Crit Care Clin 28 (2012) 301–321

doi:10.1016/j.ccc.2011.10.016

0749-0704/12/$ – see front matter © 2012 Elsevier Inc. All rights reserved.

acute elevations in afterload, the unconditioned RV suffers an abrupt decrease in stroke volume. Although an increase in RV end-diastolic volume (RVEDV) may transiently improve stroke volume through the Frank-Starling mechanism, additional increases in RVEDV further reduce global cardiac output due to RV ischemia, tricuspid regurgitation, and ventricular interdependence. The sum result of progressive pulmonary hypertension and RV failure is decreased RV stroke volume, increased RVEDV, and decreased cardiac output, resulting in the clinical presentation of systemic venous congestion and cardiogenic shock. Based on RV function and in order of decreasing risk of adverse outcomes, recent guidelines have defined high-risk PE as that which results in frank shock, with a sustained systolic blood pressure less than 90 mmHg or requiring vasopressor support. Intermediate-risk (or submassive) PE defines those with preserved blood pressure but with evidence of right heart strain or ischemia. Finally, low-risk PE occurs in those patients with neither shock nor evidence of RV dysfunction.[12,13]

Risk stratification in acute PE has been investigated by a number of techniques including clinical scoring systems, laboratory measurements (biomarkers), and imaging studies. Although the individual studies of acute PE risk stratification vary significantly in design, they all are based on knowledge of patient comorbidities and the presence of RV dysfunction. These modalities have been used in isolation and, more recently, compared and studied in combination. Whereas no risk stratification technique has clearly proved superior to the others, a familiarity with these methodologies, combined with an awareness of local test availability, can allow one to estimate prognosis for an individual patient and direct treatment appropriately.

This article reviews the following methods of acute PE risk stratification:

1. Patient characteristics and clinical scoring systems
2. Biomarkers (natriuretic peptides and cardiac troponins)
3. Imaging studies (echocardiography and computed tomographic pulmonary angiography [CTPA]).

PATIENT CHARACTERISTICS AND CLINICAL SCORING SYSTEMS

Patient characteristics that have been associated with worse prognosis after an acute PE have been consistent across most investigations. In a large multicenter cohort of patients from the United States and Europe (the International Cooperative Pulmonary Embolism Registry [ICOPER]) the following demographics and preexisting conditions were independently associated with increased all-cause 3-month mortality: age over 70 years, cancer, congestive heart failure, and chronic obstructive pulmonary disease.[4] Likewise, in other United States and European cohorts, increasing age, a history of congestive heart failure, and cancer were found to increase the risk of adverse outcomes after an acute PE.[2,14,15] In addition to patient characteristics, signs and symptoms at presentation convey prognostic information. In the ICOPER registry, a systolic blood pressure less than 90 mmHg conferred a three-fold increase risk of death at 90 days.[4] Similarly, another study found that shock (systolic blood pressure <90 mmHg or need for vasopressor) conferred a three-fold increase in risk of 30-day adverse outcome (death, secondary shock, or recurrent PE).[14] In this same study, altered mental status at presentation, which likely reflects poor cardiac output and/or hypoxia, was associated with a seven-fold increase in risk of adverse outcome.[14]

Whereas the previously described patient characteristics intuitively place patients at higher risk of adverse outcomes, several groups have attempted to more objectively classify the prognosis of patients with acute PE. In an early study, Wicki and

Table 1	
Geneva acute pulmonary embolism risk score	
Predictor	Point Score
Cancer	+2
Heart failure	+1
Previous deep vein thrombosis	+1
Systolic blood pressure <100 mmHg	+2
Pao$_2$ <8 kPa (60 mmHg) (room air)	+1
Deep vein thrombosis (by ultrasound)	+1
Total score	0–8

Low risk score is ≤2 points, whereas high risk score is ≥3.
Data from Wicki J, Perrier A, Perneger TV, et al. Predicting adverse outcome in patients with acute pulmonary embolism: a risk score. Thromb Haemost 2000;84(4):548–52.

colleagues[15] found that six factors, including three comorbidities, two laboratory findings, and the presence of a deep vein thrombosis, were able to stratify those with acute PE into low-risk and high-risk categories (**Table 1**). Patients in the low-risk group experienced a 2.2% risk of adverse outcome (mortality, recurrent thromboembolic event, or major bleeding) at 3 months. In contrast, those in the high-risk group suffered a 26.1% risk of adverse outcome. Although simple to calculate, the Wicki (or Geneva) score requires an arterial blood gas and lower extremity ultrasound examination, studies that are not often performed early in the evaluation of acute PE.

Aujesky and colleagues[3] created the pulmonary embolism severity index (PESI) in an attempt to risk-stratify patients with acute PE based on readily available clinical information. Based on a large derivation and validation cohort, the PESI established five levels of risk for 30-day mortality after acute PE based on patient demographics, comorbidities, and clinical findings (**Table 2**).[3] In the low-risk categories (class I and II), mortality at 30 days was at or lower than 3.5%, whereas those in the highest risk category (class V) had an event rate up to 24.5% (**Table 3**). Although the PESI is based on readily available clinical information, was derived from a large number of patients with a spectrum of disease severity, and has been validated in other populations, it suffers from complexity; the 11-variable computation is difficult to perform at the bedside.[16,17] Furthermore, like the Geneva score, the PESI has better negative predictive value than positive predictive value in acute PE; it identifies those at low risk but lacks specificity in identifying those at high risk of adverse events.[18] In addition, although robust in identifying those at low risk of 30-day mortality, the PESI may not be as useful in the triage of patients with acute PE. Specifically, in one study those with a low-risk PESI score (groups I–II) experienced a 14% incidence of significant adverse (although not fatal) events that would require inpatient care, including increased oxygen requirement, need for vasopressor therapy, or new arrhythmia.[19]

Despite its robust performance in predicting mortality, the impracticality of the PESI has led others to design simplified forms of PE risk stratification. Based on independent derivation and validation cohorts, a simplified PESI score was constructed of six readily available clinical features (**Table 4**).[20] Using an outcome of 30-day mortality, the positive predictive value (11% vs 11%) and negative predictive value (98% vs 99%) of the low-risk original PESI (class I–II) and simplified PESI score, respectively, were similar. Although much less complex in performance, the simplified

Table 2
Pulmonary embolism severity index

Predictor	Points Assigned
Age, per year	Age, in years
Male gender	+10
Cancer	+30
Heart failure	+10
Chronic lung disease	+10
Pulse ≥110 per minute	+20
Systolic blood pressure <100 mmHg	+30
Respiratory rate ≥30 per minute	+20
Temperature <36°C	+20
Altered mental status	+60
Arterial oxygen saturation <90%	+20

Points correspond to the following risk classes: class I ≤65, class II 66–85, class III 86–105, class IV 106–125, class V >125.
Data from Aujesky D, Obrosky DS, Stone RA, et al. Derivation and validation of a prognostic model for pulmonary embolism. Am J Resp Crit Care Med 2005;172(8):1041–6.

PESI, like the original decision tool, works better at identifying low-risk acute PE patients rather than classifying individuals at high risk of clinical worsening.

Comparison between the PESI and the Geneva score shows differences between the scoring systems. In a large independent cohort, the PESI classified 36% of patients as low-risk (class I–II), whereas the Geneva score classified 84% of patients as low-risk. Less than 1% of patients with low-risk PESI scores (class I–II) died within 30 days compared with 5.6% of low-risk Geneva score patients. The mortality in high-risk patients likewise differed, with an event rate of 10.7% for high risk PESI (class III–V) versus 15.5% for high-risk Geneva scores. Because the strength of the acute PE risk stratification systems lies in their ability to identify low-risk patients, the discriminative power of the Geneva score is inferior to that of the PESI score. That is, whereas the positive predictive value of both systems was mediocre, the negative prediction value (identifying those patients with acute PE at low risk of dying) of the PESI was superior to that of the Geneva score (99% vs 94%, respectively).[21]

Table 3
Mortality by PESI class

PESI Class	30-Day Mortality
I	≤1.6%
II	≤3.5%
III	≤7.1%
IV	≤11.4%
V	≤24.5%

Data from Aujesky D, Obrosky DS, Stone RA, et al. Derivation and validation of a prognostic model for pulmonary embolism. Am J Resp Crit Care Med 2005;172(8):1041–6.

Table 4	
Simplified pulmonary embolism severity index	
Predictor	**Points Assigned**
Age >80 years	1
History of cancer	1
History of chronic cardiopulmonary disease	1
Pulse ≥110 per minute	1
Systolic blood pressure <100 mmHg	1
Arterial oxygen saturation <90%	1

Low risk = 0 points; high risk = 1 or more points.
Data from Jimenez D, Aujesky D, Moores L, et al. Simplification of the pulmonary embolism severity index for prognostication in patients with acute symptomatic pulmonary embolism. Arch Intern Med 2010;170(15):1383–9.

BIOMARKERS

Biomarkers have emerged as promising tools through which patients with acute PE can be risk-stratified. The appeal of biomarkers lies in their wide availability irrespective of location or time of the day, generally quick response from the clinical lab, and noninvasive nature. The downside of biomarkers is that they provide only indirect evidence of RV function. Moreover, whereas they are generally reported or regarded as "positive" or "negative," in reality biomarkers are measured across a continuum; both the selection of a test cut point (the demarcation between positive and negative) and the impact of other comorbidities on test characteristics are not inconsequential details that are generally unknown to the practicing intensivist. Therefore, before using biomarkers to direct individual patient care, critical care physicians should have an understanding of the physiologic factors that influence biomarker performance and of the negative and positive predictive values of a given biomarker test result.

Natriuretic Peptides

Natriuretic peptides are a family of peptides released by the heart in response to volume overload; they collectively mediate vasodilation, natriuresis, and diuresis. In response to stretch, the cells of the ventricular myocardium will synthesize probrain natriuretic peptide. This peptide is subsequently cleaved to the biologically active brain natriuretic peptide (BNP) and the inactive amino terminal fragment (NT-proBNP).[22] Both BNP and NT-proBNP can be measured clinically and have been validated as diagnostic and prognostic markers of ventricular stretch in multiple conditions, including congestive heart failure, pulmonary hypertension, and acute PE.[22] Whereas both BNP and NT-proBNP are used in clinical practice, they have biological differences and the measured levels are not interchangeable. In particular, BNP has a shorter half-life (20 minutes) than NT-proBNP (1–2 hours). In addition, the latter is a more stable peptide and is less sensitive to changes in temperature or delays in testing.[23]

Both BNP and NT-proBNP have been extensively investigated as prognostic markers in acute PE. In an early study, ten Wolde and colleagues[24] demonstrated in a prospective cohort of normotensive acute PE patients that those who died within 90 days had a significantly increased BNP level at the time of diagnosis compared with those patients who did not die in follow-up (245 pg/mL vs 30 pg/mL, respectively). In addition, using a cut point of 75 pg/mL, these investigators reported that BNP had a positive predictive value of PE-related mortality of 17%, whereas the negative predictive value for death was 99%.[24] As will be seen for most of the prognostic markers for acute PE, the investigators noted that BNP was able to identify those at low risk of adverse outcomes but did not have good specificity (many false-positives) in identifying those who were likely to die from their PE.

In a similar early study, Kucher and colleagues[25] investigated the prognostic capabilities of NT-proBNP in a prospective cohort of acute PE patients. In those suffering an adverse event (defined as a combined end point of in-hospital death or need for escalation of care, including cardiopulmonary resuscitation, mechanical ventilation, vasopressor, or thrombolysis), NT-proBNP was significantly higher compared with those who did not experience an adverse event (median of 4250 pg/mL vs 121 pg/mL, respectively). An NT-proBNP cut point of 500 pg/mL yielded a negative predictive value for adverse outcome of 97% with a corresponding positive predictive value of adverse outcome of 45%.[25]

A separate prospective study of normotensive acute PE patients found similar results. Kostrubiec and colleagues[26] reported that an NT-proBNP value of 600 pg/mL had a negative and positive predictive value for both all-cause mortality at 40 days of 100% and 21%, respectively. In a separate study, this same group investigated the prognostic implications of NT-proBNP trends over the first 24 hours after an acute PE. As in the aforementioned study, an NT-proBNP value over 600 pg/mL had a 100% negative predictive value for death within 30 days, with a corresponding positive predictive value for mortality of 21%. However, in those patients with an NT-proBNP value over 600 pg/mL at admission and in whom the absolute NT-proBNP value did not decrease by at least 50% in the in the first 24 hours, the positive predictive value for death increased to 27%. In the same study, the positive predictive value for death in those in whom the admission value of NT-proBNP was over 7500 pg/mL increased from 46% to 61% if the absolute value of NT-proBNP did not decrease by 50% in the first 24 hours of admission.[27] The investigators postulate that in those with acute PE a persistently elevated natriuretic peptide signifies ongoing RV dysfunction and confers an increase in mortality.

In addition to the serial measurement of natriuretic peptides, the initial measurement of natriuretic peptide in temporal relation to the acute PE event may influence prognostic properties. Specifically, natriuretic peptides are minimally stored in normal myocardium and need to be transcribed and translated in response to ventricular stretch.[22] Theoretically, patients who present very early in the course of an acute PE, before the cellular machinery has had time to synthesize natriuretic peptide, may have deceptively low levels of BNP or NT-proBNP. Klok and colleagues[28] investigated this hypothesis in a post hoc analysis of a prospective acute PE cohort. Stratifying patients by the time from the start of symptoms to presentation, they found no difference in NT-proBNP values with regard to outcomes, even in those who presented within 6 hours of symptom onset. The investigators concluded that NT-proBNP (at a threshold of 600 pg/mL) could be used to risk-stratify patients with acute PE, regardless of the acuity of symptom onset.[28]

In a well-done metaanalysis, Lega and colleagues[29] summarized the available literature on natriuretic peptide use in acute PE. Overall, 52% of patients in the 23 collated studies had an elevated natriuretic peptide at presentation. Moreover, an elevated natriuretic peptide level, either BNP or NT-proBNP, conferred an independent risk of all-cause mortality, acute-PE related mortality, and serious adverse event. Specifically, an elevated BNP conferred a 5.4-fold increase in risk of mortality, whereas an increased NT-proBNP was associated with a 9.9-fold increased risk of death. They also reported that in those with both low natriuretic peptide and cardiac troponin levels at presentation that the rates of all-cause and acute PE–specific mortality were extremely low (0.2% and 0%, respectively).[29] In a different systematic review of the same literature, Cavallazzi and colleagues[30] reported that a BNP cutoff level of 100 pg/mL resulted in a positive and negative likelihood ratio of 1.7 and 0.27, respectively, for in-hospital mortality after an acute PE. Likewise, using an NT-proBNP cutoff level of 600 pg/mL yielded a positive and negative likelihood ratio of 1.45 and 0.09, respectively.[30]

Cardiac Troponins

Like natriuretic peptides, cardiac troponins have been investigated as prognostic indicators in acute PE. Troponins, both the I and T subunits, are sensitive markers of myocardial cell injury. In acute PE, myocardial ischemia and infarction probably play a role in troponin release.[31] In an early investigation in patients with acute PE, a troponin T (TnT) value of 0.01 ng/mL had a 91% negative predictive value for adverse outcomes (in-hospital death or clinical deterioration); the corresponding positive predictive value was 55%.[25] In another investigation, Janata and colleagues[32] prospectively assessed the prognostic value of TnT in patients with acute PE. They found that TnT levels were higher in those who died during their hospitalization (0.18 ng/mL vs <0.01 ng/mL in survivors) and that a TnT cutoff value of 0.09 ng/mL had a negative predictive value of 99% for short-term mortality (with a corresponding positive predictive value of 34%).[32]

Although generally assessed at the time of presentation in acute PE, cardiac troponins are followed serially in those with acute myocardial infarction. Pruszczyk and colleagues[33] investigated the time course of TnT elevation in those with acute PE. In a prospective cohort, they found that whereas 50% of normotensive patients with acute PE were found to have an elevated TnT, 5% of these patients had an initial TnT that was normal; only on subsequent (every 6 hours analysis) tests did the TnT increase. Like the earlier studies, elevated TnT was associated with a worse prognosis. In this report, 25% of those with an elevated TnT (>0.01 ng/mL) died during the hospitalization compared with no patient with a TnT value less than 0.01 ng/mL.[33]

In a recent metaanalysis, Becattini and colleagues[34] analyzed the body of literature reporting on the prognostic usefulness of cardiac troponins in acute PE. In a summary of 20 studies, they reported that 20% of patients with elevated troponins died, compared with 3.7% of patients with normal troponin levels. A high level of either TnT or troponin I (TnI) conferred a five-fold increased risk of short-term death.[34] The investigators noted that there were a multitude of different troponin assays and selected cut points used in the included reports, although results were generally consistent across studies. Most studies included in the metaanalysis defined an elevated troponin as any value that was above the upper limit of normal for the individual troponin assay. In particular, definitions for elevated TnI centered around 0.1 to 0.4 ng/mL, whereas definitions for elevated TnT were clustered around 0.01 to 0.04 ng/mL.[34]

Other Biomarkers

Although natriuretic peptides and cardiac troponins have been the most well-studied biomarkers in acute PE, several other markers have been reported. Heart-type fatty acid binding protein (H-FABP) is a cytosolic protein present in cardiac myocytes that diffuses out of injured myocardium more quickly than do cardiac troponins. Several groups have reported that H-FABP, like cardiac troponins, has a good negative predictive value for adverse outcomes in patients with acute PE.[35,36] In particular, an

H-FABP value of 6 ng/mL conferred a 99% negative prediction for complicated 30-day outcome (death, need for resuscitation, intubation, or vasopressor); the corresponding positive predictive value was 28%.[36]

Using a much more widely available biomarker, Scherz and colleagues[37] recently reported that hyponatremia is an adverse prognostic marker in those with acute PE. In this large prospective cohort, patients with presenting sodium value over 135 mmol/L, 130–135 mmol/L, and less than 130 mmol/L had corresponding 30-day mortalities of 8%, 14%, and 29%. Those patients with hyponatremia were older, had more comorbidities, and were more likely to be in PESI risk class IV to V compared with those with normal sodium values. After adjustment for patient demographics and PESI risk score, hyponatremia (sodium <130 mmol/L) remained an independent predictor of death (odds ratio 3.3, 95%; confidence interval 2.5–4.3, compared with those with normal sodium values). The investigators postulate that hyponatremia is a marker of neurohormonal activation and nonosmotic release of vasopressin consequent to poor cardiac output.[37]

Biomarker Comparison

In an effort to assess biomarker performance in the same populations, several groups have undertaken simultaneous comparison of the biomarkers mentioned earlier. Kostrubiec and colleagues[26] performed a single-center prospective comparison of NT-proBNP and TnT in consecutive normotensive patients with acute PE in predicting all-cause mortality at 40 days. In this cohort, receiver operating characteristic curve analysis showed that a TnT value greater than 0.07 ng/mL was the best cut point, with a sensitivity and specificity for all-cause mortality of 60% and 89%, respectively.

Likewise, an elevated NT-proBNP was also a significant predictor of mortality; an NT-proBNP value greater than 7600 pg/mL demonstrated sensitivity and specificity for all-cause mortality of 60% and 86%, respectively. A lower NT-proBNP cut point of 600 pg/mL had a 100% negative predictive value for all-cause and acute PE specific mortality. The group of patients with elevated NT-proBNP (>600 pg/mL) but low TnT (<0.07 ng/mL) were at intermediate risk of death (positive predictive value for mortality = 11%), whereas those patients with elevated levels of both biomarkers (NT-proBNP >600 pg/mL and TnT >0.07 ng/ml) were at highest risk of mortality (positive predictive value for mortality = 50%).[26]

In a later multicenter prospective study, Vuilleumier and colleagues[38] investigated concurrently the prognostic properties of NT-proBNP and TnI in normotensive patients with acute PE. The combined end point in this report was requirement for intensive care unit admission, death, or readmission due to PE complication in the 30 days after the initial event. The investigators used predefined cut points of 0.09 ng/mL for TnI and 300 pg/mL for NT-proBNP. They found, like the aforementioned Kostrubiec study, that a low NT-proBNP conferred a 100% negative predictive value for adverse outcome; the corresponding positive predictive value for this NT-proBNP cut point was 20%. Using a value of 0.09 ng/mL, TnI demonstrated a negative predictive value of 91% and a positive predictive value of 25% for adverse outcomes.[38]

Overall, there is robust literature support for the prognostic capability of biomarkers, particularly natriuretic peptides and cardiac troponins, in acute PE. These proteins have excellent negative predictive value in identifying patients at low risk of suffering acute PE-related death or adverse outcome. However, none of these biomarkers have good specificity with regard to mortality or clinical decompensation. Moreover, although the literature is generally consistent, the use of different assays, cut points, and clinical definitions of adverse events across studies hinders the ability of the intensivist to apply this body of literature to bedside practice.

IMAGING STUDIES

Imaging studies provide another means of risk-stratifying those with acute PE. Transthoracic echocardiography (TTE) has been widely studied in assessing prognosis in acute PE. The advantage of TTE lies in its noninvasive nature and ability to provide direct information about RV function. However, TTE is limited by its lack of around-the-clock availability in some institutions and by inadequate ultrasound images in obese patients or in those with underlying lung disease.[39,40] Another imaging modality that has been assessed in acute PE is CTPA. The strengths of CTPA for acute PE risk assessment include the combination of both diagnostic and prognostic elements into a single study and wide availability. The disadvantages of CTPA include radiation exposure and requirement for intravenous contrast dye, both of which exclude certain patient populations. Another "imaging" study that has been examined in assessing prognosis in acute PE is electrocardiography (ECG). Findings of RV strain on ECG include right bundle branch block or an S wave in lead I combined with a Q wave and T wave inversion in lead III (S1Q3T3 pattern). Although ECG is widely available, noninvasive, and easily interpreted, ECG evidence of RV strain lacks both sensitivity and specificity in identifying RV dysfunction in the setting of acute PE and will not be discussed further.[41]

Echocardiography

Echocardiography has a long been recognized as a prognostic tool in acute PE. In an early investigation, Ribeiro and colleagues[42] hypothesized that RV systolic dysfunction as characterized by TTE at the time of diagnosis of acute PE would be a predictor of mortality. RV function was assessed by several parameters including qualitative evaluation of RV wall motion and estimated pulmonary artery systolic pressure (PASP); the latter was calculated based on the tricuspid regurgitant jet velocity and use of modified Bernoulli equation. The investigators reported that 55% of patients in their study had evidence of RV dysfunction at the time of presentation. In-hospital and 1-year mortality in those with moderate to severe echocardiographic RV dysfunction were 14% and 23%, respectively, compared with 0% and 7% in those without evidence of RV dysfunction at the time of diagnosis. Although there tended to be a higher estimated PASP in those who did as compared with those who did not die in the hospital (means of 57 ± 17 versus 47 ± 14 mmHg, respectively), there was marked overlap between the groups, making this parameter less useful clinically.[42] This early study suggested that TTE may have a role in risk assessment in those with acute PE. Although the absence of RV dysfunction at the time of presentation suggested a benign clinical course, RV dysfunction by TTE was present in a majority of patients at the time of presentation, reducing the specificity of TTE for predicting mortality. Furthermore, the use of a qualitative assessment of RV function limited the generalize ability of the results.

The International Cooperative Pulmonary Embolism Registry (ICOPER) provided a large patient dataset in which to confirm these early findings. Over 1000 patients in this registry presented with normotensive acute PE and had a TTE performed within 24 hours of presentation. In this cohort, 39% of patients had evidence of RV dysfunction, defined as qualitative RV systolic hypokinesis, at the time of diagnosis. The negative and positive predictive values for 30-day mortality of echocardiographic RV dysfunction in this study were reported to be 91% and 16%, respectively.

In a subsequent investigation, Grifoni and colleagues[43] prospectively investigated the ability of RV dysfunction as assessed by TTE to predict short-term mortality in those with acute PE.[43] In this report, RV function was considered abnormal if (1) RV dilation was present (end-diastolic diameter >3 cm or RV/left ventricular [LV] end-diastolic diameter ratio >1, both in 4-chamber view), (2) paradoxical ventricular septal systolic motion, or (3) pulmonary hypertension as measured by Doppler interrogation. In this cohort, 40% of patients presenting with normotensive acute PE had TTE evidence, as previously defined, of RV dysfunction. The negative predictive value of echocardiographic signs of RV dysfunction for in-hospital mortality in this study was 100%, as compared with a positive predictive value of 5%.[43] Although confirming the results of earlier work, particularly with regard to identifying those at low risk for adverse events, this report also established quantitative measures through which RV function could be assessed.

In another study that attempted to quantitate RV dysfunction at the time of acute PE diagnosis, Fremont and colleagues[44] retrospectively investigated the prognostic capability of the RV/LV end-diastolic diameter as assessed by TTE in parasternal or subcostal views. Using registry data on over 900 patients, these investigators found an optimal end-diastolic RV/LV diameter ratio cut point for hospital mortality of 0.9, with a sensitivity of 72% and specificity of 58%. The in-hospital mortality in those with an RV/LV ratio at or above 0.9 at the time of acute PE diagnosis was 6.6%, compared with 1.9% in those with an RV/LV ratio less than 0.9. For comparison, the mean end-diastolic RV/LV ratio for all patients in the cohort was 0.74 ± 0.27.[44]

Toosi and colleagues[45] expanded the literature on quantitative echocardiographic risk assessment in acute PE with their retrospective investigation of multiple parameters of RV function. In this multicenter cohort, RV dysfunction was assessed in multiple ways, including (1) RV/LV end-diastolic diameter greater than 1, (2) RV end-diastolic diameter greater than 3 cm, and (3) estimated PASP greater than 50 mmHg. In their cohort they found that 42% had an RV/LV end-diastolic diameter greater than 1, 60% had an end-diastolic diameter greater than 3 cm, and 47% had an estimated PASP greater than 50 mmHg. The positive and negative predictive values for in-hospital mortality for these and other markers of RV dysfunction characterized in this report are outlined in **Table 5**.

Another quantitative measurement of RV function that has been more recently described is the tricuspid annular plane systolic excursion (TAPSE). TAPSE is defined as the systolic displacement of the tricuspid annulus toward the RV apex in the longitudinal plane, as measured by M-mode echocardiography. In a failing RV or an RV contracting against an elevated pulmonary artery pressure, there is less displacement

Table 5
Echocardiographic measurement of RV dysfunction and risk of mortality in acute PE

Measurement	In-Hospital Mortality	
	Positive Predictive Value	Negative Predictive Value
Moderate-severe RV hypokinesis	18%	100%
Estimated PASP >50 mmHg	19%	97%
Peak TR velocity >3.4 m/sec	20%	97%
RV/LV end-diastolic diameter >1	17%	100%
RV end-diastolic diameter >3 cm	11%	100%
Interventricular septal flattening	14%	99%

Abbreviations: PASP, pulmonary artery systolic pressure; TR, tricuspid regurgitant jet.
Data from Toosi MS, Merlino JD, Leeper KV. Prognostic value of the shock index along with transthoracic echocardiography in risk stratification of patients with acute pulmonary embolism. Am J Cardiol 2008;101(5):700–5.

of the tricuspid annulus, and TAPSE is decreased. Mean TAPSE in healthy adults is 2.5cm, whereas a value of less than 1.8cm has been validated as a negative prognostic marker in chronic pulmonary hypertension.[46-48] In a small prospective investigation of normotensive patients with acute PE, Holley and colleagues[49] assessed the prognostic utility of TAPSE in comparison with biomarkers and more well-defined echocardiographic markers of RV dysfunction. Using the previously established TAPSE cutoff of 1.8cm, these investigators found that BNP was elevated (>90 pg/mL) in 60% of those with an abnormal TAPSE compared with 5% of those with a normal TAPSE. The mean TAPSE in those with normal BNP was 2.3cm, whereas it was 1.7cm in those with an elevated BNP. Furthermore, there was a significant correlation between a reduced TAPSE and a greater RV end-diastolic diameter and a higher RV/LV end-diastolic ratio.[49] Although small and not powered for mortality, this study suggests that TAPSE, which is an easily measured marker of RV function, could likewise be used for risk assessment in those with acute PE.

Finally, in a comparison between biomarkers and TTE in patients with normotensive acute PE, Logeart and colleagues,[50] in a blinded manner, assessed the accuracy of BNP and TnI in detecting echocardiographic RV dysfunction. RV dysfunction was classified by the presence of two or more of the following: RV/LV end-diastolic diameter greater than 0.7, hypokinesis of the RV free wall, interventricular septum flattening, tricuspid regurgitant jet velocity greater than 2.7 m/s, or inferior vena cava diameter greater than 10 mm during inspiration. The mean BNP levels in those patients with and without RV dysfunction were 497 ± 327 versus 97 ± 109 pg/mL, respectively. Likewise, the mean TnI concentrations in those with and without RV dysfunction were 0.35±0.58 versus 0.05±0.08 ng/mL. The area under the receiver operating characteristic curve for the diagnosis of echocardiographic RV dysfunction was 0.93 for BNP and 0.72 for TnI. More importantly, a BNP less than 100pg/mL had a 100% negative predictive value for RV dysfunction, whereas a TnI of less than 0.10 ng/mL had a 67% negative predictive value for RV dysfunction. A combination of both BNP greater than 100 pg/mL and a TnI greater than 0.10 ng/mL had an 80% positive predictive value for echocardiographic RV dysfunction.[50] Overall, these investigators found that an increased TnI was more specific but that an increased BNP was more sensitive for RV dysfunction as assessed by echocardiography. Moreover, using a combination of biomarkers and cut points allowed these investigators to identify clinically useful negative and positive predictive values for RV dysfunction, suggesting potential use in an algorithmic approach to PE risk stratification.

CT Pulmonary Angiography

Although CTPA is well-established as a diagnostic tool in acute PE, the prognostic capability of CTPA is less well-defined relative to that of TTE. CTPA measurements that have been investigated as potential prognostic tools in acute PE include the severity of pulmonary artery obstruction (clot burden), degree of RV strain, estimation of pulmonary artery pressure via main pulmonary artery diameter, and indirect signs of elevated pulmonary vascular resistance such as reflux of contrast media into the inferior vena cava.[51] RV strain, as measured by dilation of the RV relative to the LV, is the most characterized of the CTPA prognostic parameters. Estimation of clot burden is a potentially useful prognostic tool, but the scoring systems are too complex to be used in everyday clinical practice.[52,53] The other parameters, including pulmonary artery size and contrast reflux, have not been found to be reliable criteria for PE severity.[51]

One of the early studies assessing the prognostic role of RV enlargement on CTPA in acute PE was published by Quiroz and colleagues.[54] In this retrospective analysis the RV and LV diameters were measured by identifying the maximal distance between the endocardium and the interventricular septum, perpendicular to the long axis of the heart. These measurements were taken from both the axial view and the reconstructed four-chamber view. A ratio of RV/LV diameter of greater than 0.9 was selected as the cut point, based on receiver operating characteristic curve analysis. In the axial plane analysis there was no difference in the proportion of patients with an elevated RV/LV ratio between those who suffered an adverse event (death or escalation of care) (RV/LV >0.9 in 71%) and those who did not suffer an adverse event (RV/LV >0.9 in 72%). However, an elevated RV/LV ratio was an adverse prognostic marker in the analysis of the reconstructed four-chamber views. Specifically, an elevated RV/LV ratio was more common in patients with adverse events (RV/LV >0.9 in 80%) than in those without adverse events (RV/LV >0.9 in 51%).[54]

In a subsequent and larger study, the same investigators reported the association between reconstructed four-chamber view RV/LV ratio from CTPA and mortality.[55] In this cohort, 64% of patients with acute PE had an RV/LV ratio greater than 0.9. The 30-day mortality rate was 16% in those with an elevated RV/LV ratio (>0.9), whereas those with a low RV/LV ratio experienced only an 8% 30-day mortality. The median RV/LV ratio was 1.0 in those who died and 0.95 in those who did not die. The positive and negative predictive for 30-day mortality for an RV/LV ratio greater than 0.9 were 16% and 92%, respectively.[55] However, the utility of RV diameter on CTPA in estimating prognosis has not been consistent.

Araoz and colleagues[56] evaluated the prognostic significance of three different CTPA measurements—ventricular septal bowing, quantitative clot burden, and RV/LV ratio in the axial plan—in a large single-center retrospective study. The investigators reported that in this cohort of over 1000 patients with acute PE, none of the three CTPA measures were consistently associated with 30-day mortality. Ventricular septal bowing (a subjective assessment of the septum bowing toward the LV) was a specific, albeit insensitive, marker for mortality for some radiologists, although the high interobserver variability limited the usefulness of this measurement.[56]

In another large multicenter retrospective study of over 500 patients with acute PE, RV strain as defined as an RV/LV ratio greater than 1 in axial images was associated with 30-day mortality.[57] In this study, 30% of patients with acute PE had an elevated RV/LV ratio on CTPA. Those with an elevated RV/LV ratio were more likely to have a PESI score greater than 3 (33% vs 22%) and suffered greater 30-day mortality (12% vs 5%) than those who did not have an elevated RV/LV ratio, respectively. Furthermore, within each PESI risk class, those patients with an elevated RV/LV ratio (>1) had significantly higher mortality than those patients who did not have an elevated RV/LV ratio.[57] Contrary to this report, a retrospective review of the Prospective Investigation of Pulmonary Embolism Diagnosis II database found that there was no difference in mortality between patients with and without RV enlargement (defined as an RV/LV ratio >1 in the axial plane) on CTPA.[58]

Despite the inability of CTPA measurements to reliably estimate prognosis in those with acute PE in isolation, several groups have investigated the correlation between CTPA findings and other prognostic factors. Vuilleumier and colleagues[59] showed in a prospective cohort of normotensive acute PE patients that those with a CTPA RV/LV ratio greater than 1 (in reconstructed four-chamber view) had significantly higher median BNP (170 vs 36 pg/mL), NT-proBNP (1369 vs 171 pg/mL), and TnI (0.032 vs 0 ng/mL) levels than those who did not have an elevated RV/LV ratio.[59]

Seon and colleagues[53] compared various CTPA measurements with echocardiographic RV dysfunction, defined as RV hypokinesis or RV/LV ratio greater than 1 in four-chamber view. In this report, those patients with RV dysfunction by TTE had significantly higher CTPA RV/LV ratios (1.51±0.38) compared with those who did not

Table 6
Comparison of CTPA and biomarkers in predicting mortality in those with normotensive acute PE

	CTPA RV/LV Ratio >1	Elevated TnT (>0.09 ng/mL)	Elevated NT-proBNP (>600 pg/mL)
Positive Predictive Value	16%	30%	29%
Negative Predictive Value	98%	93%	99%
Proportion Classified as High-Risk	57%	9%	28%
Proportion Classified as Low-Risk	43%	91%	72%

Data from Klok FA, Van Der Bijl N, Eikenboom HC, et al. Comparison of CT assessed right ventricular size and cardiac biomarkers for predicting short-term clinical outcome in normotensive patients suspected of having acute pulmonary embolism. J Thromb Haemost 2010;8(4):853–6.

have echocardiographic RV dysfunction (1.05 ± 0.27) (in axial view). Other CTPA measurements were also more frequent/higher in those with RV dysfunction by TTE, including clot burden, interventricular septal bowing toward the LV, and contrast regurgitation into the inferior vena cava.[53] None of these findings, however, were sensitive or specific enough to be clinically useful in isolation.

Finally, Klok and colleagues[60] prospectively assessed the ability of both CTPA and biomarkers to predict short-term mortality (6-week) in patients presenting with normotensive acute PE. In this study all patients underwent CTPA and had RV/LV ratio measured in reconstructed four-chamber view, with an RV/LV ratio greater than 1 considered abnormal. Concurrently, patients also had TnT and NT-proBNP levels determined. The resultant positive and negative predictive values for mortality are listed in **Table 6**. Although all the prognostic markers had similar negative predictive values, none had sufficient ability to identify those at high risk of mortality (low positive predictive values). A combination of CTPA RV/LV ratio greater than 1 and an elevated NT-proBNP level (>600 pg/mL) still only had a positive predictive value of 42% for mortality.[60]

Clearly, the lack of consistent findings currently limits the ability to assess prognosis by CTPA measurements alone in those with acute PE. The discordant results of the available literature likely reflect different study populations (some reports include only normotensive patients whereas others include all patients), differences in technique (axial vs reconstructed four-chamber views, different definitions of RV strain), and interobserver variability in image interpretation. However, there does seem to be a correlation between other prognostic factors in acute PE, including TTE and biomarkers, and CTPA findings. Given the ubiquity of CTPA in the diagnosis of acute PE, future work should continue to define valid and reliable CTPA prognostic features of acute PE.

ACUTE PE RISK STRATIFICATION IN PRACTICE

Recent guidelines from both American and European societies recommend risk stratification be an integral part in the evaluation and management of patients with acute PE.[13,61] Whereas these acute PE practice guidelines emphasize the prognostic utility of clinical risk prediction scores, biomarkers, and imaging studies, they do not indicate which method, if any, is the preferred means of risk stratification. Moreover, with the exception of a recently published scientific statement (**Table 7**),[12] most guidelines do not suggest or endorse particular cut points for any of the available

Table 7
American Heart Association definitions of RV dysfunction or necrosis in normotensive acute PE

Risk Stratification Test	Recommended Cut Point
Natriuretic Peptide	BNP >90 pg/mL NT-proBNP >500 pg/mL
Cardiac Troponin	TnT >0.1 ng/mL TnI >0.4 ng/mL
Transthoracic Echocardiography	Apical four-chamber view RV/LV ratio >0.9 Qualitative RV systolic dysfunction
CT Chest Pulmonary Angiography	Reconstructed four-chamber view RV/LV ratio >0.9
Electrocardiogram	New complete or incomplete right bundle branch block Anteroseptal ST elevation or depression Anteroseptal T wave inversion

Data from Jaff MR, McMurtry MS, Archer SL, et al. Management of massive and submassive pulmonary embolism, iliofemoral deep vein thrombosis, and chronic thromboembolic pulmonary hypertension: a scientific statement from the American Heart Association. Circulation 2011;123(16):1788–830.

prognostic modalities or outline specific test combinations or algorithms to denote elevated risk; the lack of detail results from scant literature on which to make specific practice recommendations.

In an attempt to address this need, several studies have recently attempted to determine the prognostic value of various risk stratification tests used in combination. Binder and colleagues[62] hypothesized that NT-proBNP testing, in combination with TTE, may increase the prognostic value of either test in isolation and define low-, intermediate-, and high-risk patient groups. In this prospective multicenter study, all patients with acute PE underwent biomarker and TTE testing at admission. The primary outcome was complicated in-hospital course defined as death or requirement for thrombolysis, vasopressors, intubation, or cardiopulmonary resuscitation. RV dysfunction by TTE was defined as an end-diastolic diameter greater than 3 cm, whereas elevated NT-proBNP was defined as greater than 1000 pg/mL. The investigators reported that NT-proBNP had a negative and positive predictive value of 95% and 25%, respectively, for the primary end point. Of note, 54% of patients in this study had an elevated NT-proBNP. Although confirming earlier work that natriuretic peptides are capable of ruling out adverse outcomes, by itself NT-proBNP was not useful in identifying patients at high risk of clinical deterioration.

The investigators next sought to identify high-risk patients by combining NT-proBNP levels with TTE. They found that although patients with elevated NT-proBNP frequently had RV dysfunction by TTE, it was rare for a patient with normal NT-proBNP to have echocardiographic evidence of RV dysfunction (2% of subjects). They therefore defined three groups of risk: (1) patients with low NT-proBNP levels, (2) patients with high NT-proBNP but normal RV function by TTE, and (3) patients with elevated NT-proBNP and RV dysfunction by TTE. The incidence of complicated hospital outcomes in these three groups were 5%, 14%, and 37%, respectively. The investigators performed a similar analysis with TnT but found troponin to be an insensitive marker of RV dysfunction by TTE, reducing its value as a first line screening test.[62]

The results of this work suggest a possible algorithm for acute PE risk stratification, in which a readily available biomarker could be used to quickly identify those at low risk for adverse outcomes and obviate the need for additional testing. Those in whom the screening test was positive could undergo further risk stratification with TTE, the results of which further defined risk of clinical deterioration.

In a subsequent study (the prognostic factors for pulmonary embolism [PREP] study) Sanchez and colleagues[14] likewise sought to establish the additional prognostic value of echocardiography and biomarkers in risk-stratifying patients with acute PE. In this multicenter prospective observational cohort, all patients underwent TTE and had TnI, BNP, and NT-proBNP measured at admission. The primary outcome was 30-day mortality, cardiogenic shock, or recurrent thromboembolism. Similar to prior investigations, certain clinical factors (history of cancer, altered mental status, tachycardia, and hypotension) portended a worse prognosis; likewise, those patients who suffered adverse events had higher levels of natriuretic peptides and TnI and greater RV/LV end-diastolic diameter ratios by TTE. Similar to the PESI score, the investigators used the outcome data from this cohort to construct a risk score for 30-day adverse events, based on factors found to be significant predictors in multivariable regression models (**Table 8**). Unlike the PESI score, this score (PREP score) incorporated biomarker (BNP) and TTE (RV/LV ratio) results to estimate prognosis. The risk of adverse events in patients in the low-risk group (class I) was less than 5%, whereas for patients in the intermediate group (class II) it was 5% to 30%. Those patients in the highest risk group (class III) had a predicted rate of adverse events in 30 days of greater than30%.[14] Although novel in that this risk score incorporated both clinical, biomarker, and imaging factors known to influence prognosis, this new risk stratification score has not been compared with the PESI risk index itself.

A proposed risk stratification algorithm for acute PE is shown in **Fig. 1**. This algorithm incorporates many of the findings previously described, including the use of clinical, biomarker, and TTE information. As described earlier, outcomes in acute PE are predicated on both patient comorbidities and the degree of RV dysfunction; the

Table 8
PREP risk score

Prognostic Factor	Categories	Points
Altered Mental Status	No	0
	Yes	10
Cardiogenic Shock	No	0
	Yes	6
Cancer	No	0
	Yes	6
BNP (pg/mL)	<100	0
	100–249	1
	250–499	2
	500–999	4
	>1000	8
TTE RV/LV Ratio	0.2–0.49	0
	0.5–0.74	3
	0.75–1.00	5
	1.00–1.25	8
	≥1.25	11

Class I (low risk) is ≤6 points; class II (intermediate risk) is 7–17 points; class III (high risk) is ≥18 points.
Data from Sanchez O, Trinquart L, Caille V, et al. Prognostic factors for pulmonary embolism: The prep study, a prospective multicenter cohort study. Am J Respir Crit Care Med 2010;181(2):168–73.

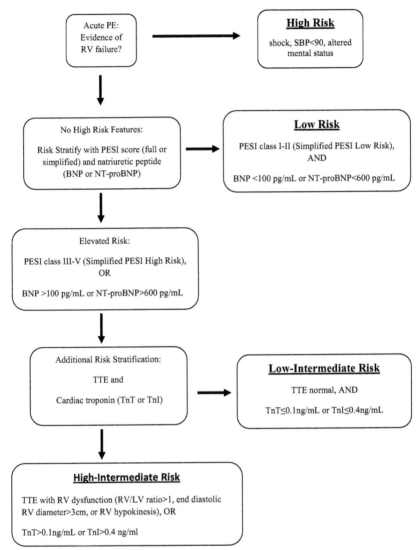

Fig. 1. Proposed acute PE risk-stratification algorithm. SBP, systolic blood pressure.

former are generally fixed, whereas the latter may be amenable to medical intervention. Risk stratification in acute PE should not only estimate likelihood of adverse events but also identify those in whom specific levels of care or therapies may improve prognosis. The proposed algorithm attempts to fulfill both these requirements through the use of clinical risk prediction scores and a stepwise approach to assessing RV function that avoids unnecessary testing. Patients who present in shock or with other associated high-risk features, such as hypotension or altered mental status, are at significant risk of death and should be considered for intensive care unit admission and possible thrombolytic therapy.[12,61] Patients in the low-risk group, those with benign clinical risk scores and no evidence by screening natriuretic peptide of RV dysfunction, are unlikely to suffer short-term complications and may be treated with conventional anticoagulation.[61] Patients in the intermediate-risk groups, with either significant comorbidities or evidence of RV dysfunction, are at elevated risk of complications and should be treated as inpatients. In particular, those with evidence of myocardial ischemia (positive troponin) or RV dysfunction by TTE—the high-intermediate risk group—may quickly decompensate and should be cared for in a higher acuity environment; the use of thrombolytics in this latter group remains controversial and the subject of ongoing investigation.[12] The course of those in the low-intermediate risk group is dictated more by underlying comorbidities and, although warranting a higher level of care, are less amenable to specific acute PE-related treatments.

SUMMARY

Risk stratification is an integral component of the diagnostic approach to acute PE. Outcomes in acute PE are dictated both by patient factors, including age and comorbidities, and the hemodynamic consequences of pulmonary thromboembolism, specifically the presence or absence of RV dysfunction. There are abundant studies describing the tools available to critical care physicians to estimate risk in acute PE, including clinical risk prediction scores, biomarkers, and imaging tests. Biomarkers, including natriuretic peptides and cardiac troponins, and TTE have clearly demonstrated prognostic value in acute PE. The former are readily available but provide only indirect evidence of RV function; the latter directly images the RV, although many intensivists will not have immediate access to echocardiography. CTPA could be a useful prognostic tool because it is already widely used for diagnosis of acute PE. Unfortunately, the literature on risk stratification based on CTPA variables is inconsistent; more work is needed before relying on this imaging technique. Although often studied in isolation, there is a growing body of literature on the combination of risk stratification methods to better estimate outcomes. Although the negative predictive value for adverse events is high for many risk prediction tools, the positive predictive value for all of these investigations, except those in patients who present in cardiogenic shock, remains low.

For intensivists, one of the main reasons to undertake risk stratification in those with acute PE is to weigh the need for thrombolytic therapy, an intervention with significant potential risk. Clearly, risk stratification techniques with greater positive predictive value for clinical deterioration or death would be desirable. Ongoing studies should continue to improve on risk assessment and therefore allow critical care physicians to more closely align intensity of therapeutic intervention with chance of adverse outcome in patients with acute PE.

REFERENCES

1. Agnelli G, Becattini C. Acute pulmonary embolism. N Engl J Med 2010;363(3): 266–74.
2. Spencer FA, Goldberg RJ, Lessard D, et al. Factors associated with adverse outcomes in outpatients presenting with pulmonary embolism: he Worcester Venous Thromboembolism Study. Circ Cardiovasc Qual Outcomes 2010;3(4):390–4.
3. Aujesky D, Obrosky DS, Stone RA, et al. Derivation and validation of a prognostic model for pulmonary embolism. Am J Resp Crit Care Med 2005;172(8):1041–6.
4. Goldhaber SZ, Visani L, De Rosa M. Acute pulmonary embolism: clinical outcomes in the International Cooperative Pulmonary Embolism Registry (ICOPER). Lancet 1999; 353(9162):1386–9.

5. Kasper W, Konstantinides S, Geibel A, et al. Management strategies and determinants of outcome in acute major pulmonary embolism: results of a multicenter registry. J Am Coll Cardiol 1997;30(5):1165–71.

6. Buller HR, Davidson BL, Decousus H, et al. Subcutaneous fondaparinux versus intravenous unfractionated heparin in the initial treatment of pulmonary embolism. N Engl J Med 2003;349(18):1695–702.

7. Simonneau G, Sors H, Charbonnier B, et al. A comparison of low-molecular-weight heparin with unfractionated heparin for acute pulmonary embolism. The THESEE Study Group. Tinzaparin ou Heparin Standard: Evaluations dans l'Embolie Pulmonaire. N Engl J Med 1997;337(10):663–9.

8. Vieillard-Baron A, Page B, Augarde R, et al. Acute cor pulmonale in massive pulmonary embolism: incidence, echocardiographic pattern, clinical implications and recovery rate. Intensive Care Med 2001;27(9):1481–6.

9. Goldhaber SZ, Elliott CG. Acute pulmonary embolism: part I; epidemiology, pathophysiology, and diagnosis. Circulation 2003;108(22):2726–9.

10. Chin KM, Kim NH, Rubin LJ. The right ventricle in pulmonary hypertension. Coron Artery Dis 2005;16(1):13–8.

11. Haddad F, Doyle R, Murphy DJ, et al. Right ventricular function in cardiovascular disease, part II: pathophysiology, clinical importance, and management of right ventricular failure. Circulation 2008;117(13):1717–31.

12. Jaff MR, McMurtry MS, Archer SL, et al. Management of massive and submassive pulmonary embolism, iliofemoral deep vein thrombosis, and chronic thromboembolic pulmonary hypertension: a scientific statement from the American Heart Association. Circulation 2011;123(16):1788–830.

13. Torbicki A, Perrier A, Konstantinides S, et al. Guidelines on the diagnosis and management of acute pulmonary embolism: The Task Force for the Diagnosis and Management of Acute Pulmonary Embolism of the European Society of Cardiology (ESC). Eur Heart J 2008;29(18):2276–315.

14. Sanchez O, Trinquart L, Caille V, et al. Prognostic factors for pulmonary embolism: The prep study, a prospective multicenter cohort study. Am J Respir Crit Care Med 2010;181(2):168–73.

15. Wicki J, Perrier A, Perneger TV, et al. Predicting adverse outcome in patients with acute pulmonary embolism: a risk score. Thromb Haemost 2000;84(4):548–52.

16. Aujesky D, Roy PM, Le Manach CP, et al. Validation of a model to predict adverse outcomes in patients with pulmonary embolism. Eur Heart J 2006;27(4):476–81.

17. Chan CM, Woods C, Shorr AF. The validation and reproducibility of the pulmonary embolism severity index. J Thromb Haemost 2010;8(7):1509–14.

18. Aujesky D, Obrosky DS, Stone RA, et al. A prediction rule to identify low-risk patients with pulmonary embolism. Arch Intern Med 2006;166(2):169–75.

19. Hariharan P, Takayesu JK, Kabrhel C. Association between the pulmonary embolism severity index (PESI) and short-term clinical deterioration. Thromb Haemost 2011; 105(4):706–11.

20. Jimenez D, Aujesky D, Moores L, et al. Simplification of the pulmonary embolism severity index for prognostication in patients with acute symptomatic pulmonary embolism. Arch Intern Med 2010;170(15):1383–9.

21. Jimenez D, Yusen RD, Otero R, et al. Prognostic models for selecting patients with acute pulmonary embolism for initial outpatient therapy. Chest 2007;132(1):24–30.

22. Daniels LB, Maisel AS. Natriuretic peptides. J Am Coll Cardiol 2007;50(25):2357–68.

23. Ordonez-Llanos J, Collinson PO, Christenson RH. Amino-terminal pro-B-type natriuretic peptide: analytic considerations. Am J Cardiol 2008;101(3A):9–15.

24. ten Wolde M, Tulevski II, Mulder JW, et al. Brain natriuretic peptide as a predictor of adverse outcome in patients with pulmonary embolism. Circulation 2003;107(16): 2082–4.

25. Kucher N, Printzen G, Doernhoefer T, et al. Low pro-brain natriuretic peptide levels predict benign clinical outcome in acute pulmonary embolism. Circulation 2003; 107(12):1576–8.

26. Kostrubiec M, Pruszczyk P, Bochowicz A, et al. Biomarker-based risk assessment model in acute pulmonary embolism. Eur Heart J 2005;26(20):2166–72.

27. Kostrubiec M, Pruszczyk P, Kaczynska A, et al. Persistent NT-proBNP elevation in acute pulmonary embolism predicts early death. Clin Chim Acta 2007;382(1-2): 124–8.

28. Klok FA, van der Bijl N, Mos IC, et al. Timing of NT-pro-BNP sampling for predicting adverse outcome after acute pulmonary embolism. Thromb Haemost 2010;104(1): 189–90.

29. Lega JC, Lacasse Y, Lakhal L, et al. Natriuretic peptides and troponins in pulmonary embolism: a meta-analysis. Thorax 2009;64(10):869–75.

30. Cavallazzi R, Nair A, Vasu T, et al. Natriuretic peptides in acute pulmonary embolism: a systematic review. Intensive Care Med 2008;34(12):2147–56.

31. Kucher N, Goldhaber SZ. Cardiac biomarkers for risk stratification of patients with acute pulmonary embolism. Circulation 2003;108(18):2191–4.

32. Janata K, Holzer M, Laggner AN, et al. Cardiac troponin T in the severity assessment of patients with pulmonary embolism: cohort study. BMJ 2003;326(7384):312–3.

33. Pruszczyk P, Bochowicz A, Torbicki A, et al. Cardiac troponin T monitoring identifies high-risk group of normotensive patients with acute pulmonary embolism. Chest 2003;123(6):1947–52.

34. Becattini C, Vedovati MC, Agnelli G. Prognostic value of troponins in acute pulmonary embolism: a meta-analysis. Circulation 2007;116(4):427–33.

35. Boscheri A, Wunderlich C, Langer M, et al. Correlation of heart-type fatty acid-binding protein with mortality and echocardiographic data in patients with pulmonary embolism at intermediate risk. Am Heart J 2010;160(2):294–300.

36. Dellas C, Puls M, Lankeit M, et al. Elevated heart-type fatty acid-binding protein levels on admission predict an adverse outcome in normotensive patients with acute pulmonary embolism. J Am Coll Cardiol 2010;55(19):2150–7.

37. Scherz N, Labarere J, Mean M, et al. Prognostic importance of hyponatremia in patients with acute pulmonary embolism. Am J Respir Crit Care Med 2010;182(9): 1178–83.

38. Vuilleumier N, Le Gal G, Verschuren F, et al. Cardiac biomarkers for risk stratification in non-massive pulmonary embolism: s multicenter prospective study. J Thromb Haemost 2009;7(3):391–8.

39. Fisher MR, Criner GJ, Fishman AP, et al. Estimating pulmonary artery pressures by echocardiography in patients with emphysema. Eur Respir J 2007;30(5):914–21.

40. Arcasoy SM, Christie JD, Ferrari VA, et al. Echocardiographic assessment of pulmonary hypertension in patients with advanced lung disease. Am J Respir Crit Care Med 2003;167(5):735–40.

41. Vanni S, Polidori G, Vergara R, et al. Prognostic value of ECG among patients with acute pulmonary embolism and normal blood pressure. Am J Med 2009;122(3): 257–64.

42. Ribeiro A, Lindmarker P, Juhlin-Dannfelt A, et al. Echocardiography Doppler in pulmonary embolism: right ventricular dysfunction as a predictor of mortality rate. Am Heart J 1997;134(3):479–87.

43. Grifoni S, Olivotto I, Cecchini P, et al. Short-term clinical outcome of patients with acute pulmonary embolism, normal blood pressure, and echocardiographic right ventricular dysfunction. Circulation 2000;101(24):2817–22.
44. Fremont B, Pacouret G, Jacobi D, et al. Prognostic value of echocardiographic right/left ventricular end-diastolic diameter ratio in patients with acute pulmonary embolism: Results from a monocenter registry of 1,416 patients. Chest 2008;133(2): 358–62.
45. Toosi MS, Merlino JD, Leeper KV. Prognostic value of the shock index along with transthoracic echocardiography in risk stratification of patients with acute pulmonary embolism. Am J Cardiol 2008;101(5):700–5.
46. Forfia PR, Fisher MR, Mathai SC, et al. Tricuspid annular displacement predicts survival in pulmonary hypertension. Am J Respir Crit Care Med 2006;174(9): 1034–41.
47. Burgess MI, Mogulkoc N, Bright-Thomas RJ, et al. Comparison of echocardiographic markers of right ventricular function in determining prognosis in chronic pulmonary disease. J Am Soc Echocardiogr 2002;15(6):633–9.
48. Koestenberger M, Ravekes W, Everett AD, et al. Right ventricular function in infants, children and adolescents: reference values of the tricuspid annular plane systolic excursion (TAPSE) in 640 healthy patients and calculation of z-score values. J Am Soc Echocardiogr 2009;22(6):715–9.
49. Holley AB, Cheatham JG, Jackson JL, et al. Novel quantitative echocardiographic parameters in acute PE. J Thromb Thrombolysis 2009;28(4):506–12.
50. Logeart D, Lecuyer L, Thabut G, et al. Biomarker-based strategy for screening right ventricular dysfunction in patients with non-massive pulmonary embolism. Intensive Care Med 2007;33(2):286–92.
51. Ferretti GR, Collomb D, Ravey JN, et al. Severity assessment of acute pulmonary embolism: role of CT angiography. Semin Roentgenol 2005;40(1):25–32.
52. Qanadli SD, El Hajjam M, Vieillard-Baron A, et al. New CT index to quantify arterial obstruction in pulmonary embolism: comparison with angiographic index and echocardiography. AJR Am J Roentgenol 2001;176(6):1415–20.
53. Seon HJ, Kim KH, Lee WS, et al. Usefulness of computed tomographic pulmonary angiography in the risk stratification of acute pulmonary thromboembolism. Comparison with cardiac biomarkers. Circ J 2011;75(2):428–36.
54. Quiroz R, Kucher N, Schoepf UJ, et al. Right ventricular enlargement on chest computed tomography: prognostic role in acute pulmonary embolism. Circulation 2004;109(20):2401–4.
55. Schoepf UJ, Kucher N, Kipfmueller F, et al. Right ventricular enlargement on chest computed tomography: a predictor of early death in acute pulmonary embolism. Circulation 2004;110(20):3276–80.
56. Araoz PA, Gotway MB, Harrington JR, et al. Pulmonary embolism: prognostic CT findings. Radiology 2007;242(3):889–97.
57. Singanayagam A, Chalmers JD, Scally C, et al. Right ventricular dilation on CT pulmonary angiogram independently predicts mortality in pulmonary embolism. Respir Med 2010;104(7):1057–62.
58. Stein PD, Beemath A, Matta F, et al. Enlarged right ventricle without shock in acute pulmonary embolism: prognosis. Am J Med 2008;121(1):34–42.
59. Vuilleumier N, Righini M, Perrier A, et al. Correlation between cardiac biomarkers and right ventricular enlargement on chest CT in non massive pulmonary embolism. Thromb Res 2008;121(5):617–24.

60. Klok FA, Van Der Bijl N, Eikenboom HC, et al. Comparison of CT assessed right ventricular size and cardiac biomarkers for predicting short-term clinical outcome in normotensive patients suspected of having acute pulmonary embolism. J Thromb Haemost 2010;8(4):853–6.
61. Kearon C, Kahn SR, Agnelli G, et al. Antithrombotic therapy for venous thromboembolic disease: American College of Chest Physicians Evidence-Based Clinical Practice Guidelines (8th edition). Chest 2008;133(6 Suppl):454S–545S.
62. Binder L, Pieske B, Olschewski M, et al. N-terminal probrain natriuretic peptide or troponin testing followed by echocardiography for risk stratification of acute pulmonary embolism. Circulation 2005;112(11):1573–9.